EASY LABOR

EASY LABOR

Every Woman's Guide to
Choosing Less Pain and More Joy
During Childbirth

William Camann, M.D.,
and
Kathryn J. Alexander, M.A.

BALLANTINE BOOKS
NEW YORK

A Ballantine Books Trade Paperback Original

Copyright © 2006 by William Camann, M.D., and Kathryn J. Alexander, M.A.

Published in the United States by Ballantine Books, an imprint of The Random House Publishing Group, a division of Random House, Inc., New York.

BALLANTINE and colophon are registered trademarks of Random House, Inc.

LIBRARY OF CONGRESS CATALOGING-IN-PUBLICATION DATA
Camann, William.
Easy labor : every woman's guide to choosing less pain and more joy during childbirth / William Camann, and Kathryn Alexander.
p. cm.
Includes index.
ISBN 0-345-47663-8
1. Pregnancy. 2. Childbirth. 3. Analgesia.
I. Alexander, Kathryn. II. Title.
RG525.C313 2006
618.2—dc22 2005048141

Printed in the United States of America

www.ballantinebooks.com

9 8 7 6 5 4 3 2

Book design by Jennifer Ann Daddio

For Alexandria and Priscilla, my beautiful little girls
—K.J.A.

For Rhonda, Zac, and Andy
—W.R.C.

Acknowledgments

I would like to acknowledge and express my sincere gratitude to all of the women who have birthed their babies at the Brigham and Women's Hospital in Boston over the last twenty years. You have taught me more than any textbook ever could. My thanks also to all the anesthesiologists, nurses, obstetricians, midwives, and doulas with whom I have had the pleasure to work. You have been a source of inspiration and a model of professionalism. Finally, my gratitude to Kathi Alexander, whose tireless dedication to the research, writing, and accuracy of this book will allow the readers to make informed and intelligent decisions with regard to pain management options during childbirth.

William Camann, M.D.

First, thank you to Bill Camann. Your broadmindedness and compassion on the topic of labor-pain relief created a thoughtful, informative book that I know will help many women have the childbirth experience they desire. Your professional knowledge and experience consistently provided enlightenment, and your sense of humor always made the process enjoyable. It was truly a pleasure working with you.

Many thanks to the smartest women I know, who encouraged me when this was no more than a thought (more like an obsession), and who provided support, and sometimes boring proofreading, along the way: Dawn McKenna, Michelle M. Fisher, Elizabeth Harvey, Christina McKenna, Jean Mellott, Hope Estrada, and Susan Thomson. Affection and gratitude to Esther Miller for your skillful guidance. Thanks and love to my entire family, and to my mother, Mary Ellen Parker and her husband, Alan, and to my father, William Alexander. And finally, with much love and gratitude to my husband, Robert Bañuelos, thank you for wholeheartedly supporting me on this project from the very beginning, and for working so hard for all of the women in your life!

Kathryn J. Alexander, M.A.

Contents

Acknowledgments   vii

Introduction: A NEW PHILOSOPHY, A NEW
     APPROACH   xi

How to Read This Book: A GUIDE FOR THOSE
     WHO LIKE TO SKIP AROUND   xvii

One: CHOOSING THE BEST BIRTH
     ENVIRONMENT FOR *YOU*   3

Two: YOUR LABOR PAIN—HOW PAINFUL IS IT?
     REALLY.   24

Three: YOUR VERY NORMAL, VERY COMMON
     FEARS OF CHILDBIRTH   52

Four: FULL-THROTTLE PAIN RELIEF:
     TECHNIQUES THAT CAN *ELIMINATE* YOUR
     LABOR PAIN   72

Five: EASING THE PAIN: MEDICATIONS TO
     RELIEVE (BUT NOT ELIMINATE) YOUR PAIN   116

Six: COMPLEMENTARY AND ALTERNATIVE
APPROACHES TO LABOR-PAIN RELIEF   137

Seven: PAIN RELIEF FOR A CESAREAN DELIVERY   200

Eight: WANT TO AVOID PAINFUL SUFFERING?
SO DID THEY   214

Nine: DON'T LET THIS HAPPEN TO YOU   229

Ten: BIRTH STORIES FROM THE OTHER SIDE
OF THE STIRRUPS!   246

Eleven: HOW YOUR CAREGIVER'S ATTITUDES
CAN IMPACT YOUR CHILDBIRTH
EXPERIENCE   269

Notes   285

Further Acknowledgments   299

Index   303

A NEW PHILOSOPHY,
A NEW APPROACH

Congratulations! You're having a baby! Whether you are preparing for your first childbirth or if you are already a veteran mom, your desire for an easy labor is shared by most pregnant women. It is perfectly natural to want a safe, comfortable, and joyful childbirth.

Most women describe childbirth as one of the most beautiful, joyful, *and* painful moments of their lives. This book offers advice on how to experience less pain and more joy during childbirth by promoting the use of the best medical and non-medical pain-relief techniques.

An easy labor is a childbirth experience you *can* strive for and *can* achieve with the proper support, preparation, and access to *all* pain-relief options. It is true that many labors end up being hard, even with good preparation and support, but the fact is, an easy labor is possible.

Since the beginning of time childbirth has been an extremely painful experience. Advances made in modern medicine, combined with an increased understanding and acceptance of alternative pain-relief methods, can profoundly influence how you experience childbirth. For you, labor and delivery do not need to be associated with pain and suffering.

As director of obstetric anesthesia at the Brigham and Women's Hospital in Boston, one of the busiest maternity units in the country, I oversee the care and comfort of women during the delivery of almost ten thousand babies a year. After nearly twenty years spent providing pain relief to laboring mothers, I have observed that women who arrive *prepared, open-minded, and flexible* throughout the course of their labor and delivery seem to fare best and appear more satisfied with their childbirth experience.

The consistent observation I have made, after speaking with thousands of women and assessing their pain-relief requests, is that mothers who have prepared themselves by learning about various pain-management methods, and who have a basic understanding of the risks and benefits of medical interventions, are more confident when making choices for pain relief during labor. In the midst of the often unpredictable experience of childbirth, women who are open-minded to the use of various pain-relief options, and who remain flexible in their approach to pain management throughout the course of their labor, are more likely to have the safe and comfortable birth they desire.

As you grow closer to your due date you may be feeling a combination of excitement, relief, wonder, and concern over your impending labor and delivery. I assure you, this unusual mix of emotions is quite common for pregnant women, and the concern that typically tops the list, right up there with the health and well-being of your newborn, is the issue of pain relief during childbirth.

Women today enjoy more pain-control choices than during any other time in history. However, until recently, pain relief during childbirth was often considered an either-or proposition. Either you were going to choose to have a baby "naturally," using no medication, or you were going to use the best medical pain-relief options available, typically an epidural, to relieve pain during childbirth. Many moms discover that they have a variety of options available to them, and those options often include a combination of both medical and nonmedical (alternative) pain-control interventions. Once labor begins, many women find that their *own particular* course of labor will determine which of those options are most effective in providing a comfortable birth experience.

Women preparing for childbirth no longer have to think in terms of Lamaze *or* epidural, narcotics *or* massage. For many women the most effective pain-management strategy uses techniques from either "side of the fence." Both can offer benefits and both can help you through your labor. The ideal pain-relief approach leaves it up to you to determine, with the support of your caregivers, which of the natural and medical pain-relief options work for you throughout the course of your labor.

In this book we describe which methods of pain relief women have found to be most effective in alleviating their labor pain and which methods have been determined by women to be less effective. We also explain how the success or failure of a particular pain-relief method often depends upon a variety of factors unique to the individual woman.

DIFFERENT POINTS OF VIEW

Women have sought ways to eliminate the pain of childbirth for centuries, yet the idea of childbirth without pain continues to spark much controversy and heated debate. There are vast differences that split caregivers, childbirth advocates, and pregnant women themselves regarding what is considered the best birth experience for a woman and her newborn.

The goal of this book is to provide you with the information you will need to make confident, informed choices regarding your pain-relief preferences well before the day of your baby's birth. Once labor begins, your understanding of the pain-relief choices available will help you feel empowered to keep all of your options open and determine for yourself which pain-relief methods reflect your own values, priorities, and personal preferences.

The focus on pain-management techniques in childbirth preparation courses and popular childbirth literature has not kept pace with the reality of women's preferences on the maternity unit. In spite of the fact that today roughly 80 percent of women who give birth in a hospital choose some form of pain-relief medication during childbirth, many childbirth education courses continue to place an emphasis on promoting the use of natural childbirth strategies, avoiding whenever possible, or for as long as possible, the use of medical pain-relief options. The message often conveyed to pregnant women is that they should do all they can to learn techniques that will help them *cope* with the intense pain of childbirth. Medical pain-relief methods that can safely and effectively help women *avoid, reduce,* or *eliminate* labor pain are often understated.

THE IMPORTANCE OF LEARNING ABOUT BOTH MEDICAL AND NONMEDICAL METHODS OF LABOR-PAIN RELIEF

Some women can effectively manage their labor pain through the use of nonmedical techniques such as focused breathing, relaxation, or water immersion throughout their entire labor and delivery. But most women prefer to reduce or eliminate their labor pain through the use of medical pain relief as soon as it is safely possible. However, even these women, especially during early labor, can still benefit from using a variety of nonmedical techniques to manage their labor pain. Women who do not learn about the various nonmedical pain-management strategies are often distressed when they discover they may have to face several hours of dealing with pain before they can benefit from medical pain-relief interventions.

The popularly promoted notion that less (or no) medical pain-relief intervention is the ideal goal often collides with an unanticipated reality, when women who wish to avoid pain-relief medications or an epidural discover their labor pain is far greater than they had prepared for, and their nonmedical pain-management methods provide inadequate relief. Women who prepare for an entirely medication-free childbirth, but who do not learn about their medical pain-relief options, are faced with having to make pain-relief choices in the midst of labor without the benefit of knowledge and preparation.

In this book we provide you with information needed to both cope with the pain that cannot be avoided and reduce or eliminate your labor pain whenever safely possible, according to your own preference for pain relief.

Over the years I have worked with women who have dealt with the pain of childbirth in almost every way possible, and the differences in choice of and preference for pain relief are sometimes striking. I have seen women committed to giving birth using absolutely no medical pain relief, who endured hours of extraordinary pain during labor and delivery, and who described their birth experience as wonderful and rewarding. I have worked with women who have come into the labor and delivery room frightened and overwhelmed by their pain (and perhaps by the entire birth experience), who requested, demanded, or pleaded for pain relief and were unable to feel a sense of control and satisfaction until their pain was completely eliminated. But most often I see women who arrive on the labor and delivery unit with a strong preference for pain control, who prefer safe and effective medical pain-relief methods, combined with the successful use of nonmedical pain-management techniques.

The desire for relief of pain is one of the most basic of human instincts. The pain of childbirth is one of the most intense feelings that a woman will experience in her lifetime. We hope this book will enable you to fully understand all of your pain-relief options, and the advantages, disadvantages, risks, and benefits to you and your newborn, so you may make the choices best suited for you to enjoy an *easy labor* filled with less pain and more joy.

William Camann, M.D.

A GUIDE FOR THOSE WHO LIKE TO SKIP AROUND

We expect that you are reading this book in order to gain information about what labor feels like and how to relieve your labor pain. We hope you will read it from cover to cover, but you may also prefer to just read certain sections concerning particular aspects of pain relief. Below we have suggested specific sections of the book that may be most helpful, depending upon your particular interests or concerns.

If you are "feeling like a chicken," especially as your due date approaches, and are worried or fearful about the pain of labor and childbirth, you may find some much-needed reassurance in chapter three, "Your Very Normal, Very Common Fears of Childbirth."

If you want to know what childbirth *feels like,* because you are a first-time mom, and it seems like a virtual impossibility at this point that you will ever get that baby from point A (the womb) to point B (the world), read chapter two, "Your Labor Pain: How Painful Is It? Really."

If you want to learn about a technique that will teach you how to literally *rethink* your fears associated with childbirth, turn to the section titled "Hypnotherapy—Changing Your *Mind*

About Labor Pain," in chapter six (page 165). This formerly "alternative" approach is gaining popularity on labor and delivery units.

If you are certain you want an epidural and therefore you think you don't need to learn about any other methods, go straight to the caregiver interviews in chapter two, under "Are You Prepared?" (page 42) to hear from the experts about why your plan for an epidural may be a good one (for you), but your plan to skip over information on any other pain-relief method is *not*! Then flip to chapter six, "Complementary and Alternative Approaches to Labor-Pain Relief."

You might be wondering why a book about labor-pain relief includes information on birth philosophies that do not necessarily provide, and may even discourage, medical pain relief.

In our opinion, it is not possible to talk about pain-relief options without acknowledging the various perspectives and strongly held, often opposing, beliefs on this topic. Some women, whether they strive for a pain-free birth through the use of modern medicine, or are committed to a medication-free birth, feel that their particular approach is not supported by other women, or by caregivers, as the "correct" way to have a baby.

We hope the inclusion of differing viewpoints and information on various birth methods increases your awareness of *all* of the pain-management options available to you. The wide range of perspectives on the topic of pain relief during childbirth shared by women throughout this book underscores the highly individual and personal nature of women's choices regarding labor-pain relief.

We have used "he" or "husband" throughout the book to refer to "partner," simply for the sake of ease.

You may notice that many of the studies done in the fields of medicine and alternative medicine are conflicting and inconclusive, in part because it is difficult to conduct reliable studies on women during childbirth. Medications, techniques, and practices also change fairly quickly in the field of medicine, so a study done on a particular drug or intervention used during childbirth may not be relevant when an adjustment or change takes place and is put into use after the conclusion of the study.

Another challenge in the research of labor pain and its relief is the variable nature of the pain experienced among women. As described in chapter two, labor pain is influenced by a number of different factors, among them pelvic shape, size and position of the newborn, and the speed (or slowness) of cervical dilation. These variables among women in labor present more of a challenge to researchers trying to determine or measure a specific outcome. In addition, women's reports of their own labor pain during birth have been shown to change even two or three days after giving birth. This factor may also alter the findings of studies done on women during the process of giving birth.

For many types of labor-pain relief, whether medical or nonmedical, there is simply not a large body of solid research available from which to draw definitive conclusions. In this book we have chosen the most widely accepted, most relevant, and most recent research studies available. We hope this information will help you feel less anxious, more prepared, and better able to enjoy an *easy labor.*

EASY LABOR

One

CHOOSING THE
BEST BIRTH
ENVIRONMENT
FOR *YOU*

Your choice of birth environment is the first decision you make that determines your pain-relief options. If you know you want to use modern medical pain-relief methods, you will need to select a birth environment that can accommodate these preferences. If you are leaning more toward a natural childbirth, but would like to keep your options open, you may want to be in a birth environment that offers not only nonmedical forms of pain relief but also allows accessibility to medical pain relief, should you change your mind during labor. If you are committed to using no medical pain-relief options and do not want to be in an environment where they are frequently used, you will need to choose a birth environment that has both the physical amenities and supportive caregivers you will need to successfully give birth free of any medications, using complementary and alternative pain-management techniques.

The staff of *caregivers* available to you during labor and birth can also directly impact your pain-relief options. For instance, if you think you prefer to use an epidural but are in a hospital where the only anesthesiologist is on another unit at the time when you are in need of pain relief, this can significantly impact your birth experience. Conversely, if you prefer to delay or avoid the use of medications, a busy hospital with a high percentage of epidural usage may not be the ideal environment for you to achieve this goal.

> Pharmacologic methods (medications) should never replace personal attention and tender loving care of the woman in labor.[1]

Your birth environment and the people caring for you during your labor and delivery can dramatically impact how you will perceive your childbirth experience. By choosing the type of birth environment best for you, you are more likely to feel relaxed and comfortable when you arrive and throughout the rest of your labor and birth. If you are giving birth in the setting you desire, surrounded by people who are able to meet your needs, including your pain-management needs, you are more likely to have a satisfying "birth day."

In this chapter we:

- List the most common birth environments.
- Describe what each has to offer with regard to pain-relief options.
- Provide a description of the various professionals who may (or may not) be with you during labor and birth.
- Provide an at-a-glance comparison between hospitals and birth centers.

HOSPITALS

Most women in the United States (approximately 98 percent) give birth in a hospital. But all hospitals are not alike, and maternity units vary greatly from hospital to hospital. In addition, the size of the hospital and its maternity unit can impact the type of birth experience you have.

Reasons You May Want to Have Your Baby in a Hospital

- You want to be in a place where all or most medical pain-relief options will be available to you.
- You want to give birth in a setting that has equipment and staff ready to deal with an unlikely emergency.
- You feel more confident in a birth environment surrounded by a variety of medical professionals.
- You want a two- to four-day recovery period before returning home with your new baby.

Larger hospitals typically offer more medical pain-management options than are found in smaller (community) hospitals. Larger hospitals are more likely to have an in-house, around-the-clock anesthesiology staff readily available if you are in need of an epidural. Often, these larger hospitals have anesthesiologists who are assigned *specifically* to the maternity unit. This reduces the likelihood of delays for women in need of pain relief that must be given by the anesthesiologist.

Smaller hospitals may not have as many medical pain-relief options and may not offer epidurals twenty-four hours a day, seven days a week. If they have a limited anesthesia staff, some smaller hospitals may not offer epidurals at all. On the other hand, many of these small hospitals, as a result of not having as much "high-tech" pain relief to offer, often have staff and equipment that can successfully support the mom who prefers to use fewer or no medications throughout labor and birth. So, depending upon your own preferences, either of these settings may be right for you. But, clearly, if you desire the full-throttle pain relief of an epidural, you are more likely to find this type of pain management taking place in larger hospitals with busier maternity units.

Size of Hospital Maternity Unit and Their Epidural and Combined Spinal-Epidural Rates:

- In hospitals that deliver fifteen hundred or more babies per year, 69 percent of women use an epidural or a combined spinal-epidural.
- In hospitals that deliver five hundred to fifteen hundred babies per year, 50 percent of women use an epidural or a combined spinal-epidural.
- In hospitals that deliver less than five hundred babies per year, 40 percent of women use an epidural or combined spinal-epidural.[2]

Hospitals of all sizes are increasingly responding to women's requests for more pain-management options, including baths, showers, the use of birth balls, and the promotion of movement and positioning during labor and birth. More hospitals are encouraging, or at the very least accepting, women's choice to use doulas (described in this chapter) as their primary support people during their labor and birth.

Many hospitals throughout the country have made their birthing rooms more appealing and homelike, with the goal of helping women feel relaxed and comfortable in the unfamiliar and sometimes intimidating surroundings of a clinical setting. Even with these changes, the hospital stay (which, for most women, is their very *first* hospital stay) can make you feel like, well, like you're in a hospital! Many caregivers recommend you bring your own homelike objects of comfort that will promote a sense of familiarity and relaxation in an otherwise unfamiliar setting. You may want to bring your favorite pillow, fragrance, photos, and a radio or CD player to listen to your favorite music. If you feel more comfy in your own clothing, let the hospital staff know you would like to wear your own threads instead of their hospital gown.

Two more factors may also determine where you ultimately give birth: your insurance coverage, which may or may not cover your care at your preferred hospital, and your obstetrician's hospital affiliation. The hospital in which your obstetrician or midwife works will be the hospital where you will have your baby. If you like your obstetrician or midwife, but do not like the hospital with which he or she is affiliated, you may find you will need to switch to a doctor or midwife who works in the hospital where you want to have your baby.

ARE WOMEN WHO HAVE THEIR BABIES IN HOSPITALS SATISFIED WITH THEIR EXPERIENCE?

According to a survey of sixteen hundred women across the country:

Ninety-six percent said they were *satisfied* with the health care they received.

Ninety-four percent felt they were *treated with kindness and understanding.*

Eighty-seven percent said they were *free to make their own decisions.*[3]

THE BIRTH CENTER

Birth centers grew popular in the 1970s as an alternative to the hospital birth experience. Birth centers may also be called alternative birth centers (ABCs) or childbearing centers. According to the National Association of Childbearing Centers, "birth centers are guided by principles of prevention, sensitivity, safety, appropriate medical intervention, and cost effectiveness."[4] Birth centers, unlike hospitals, do not exist in many communities across the country and, depending on where you live, may not be an option available to you.

Reasons You May Want to Have Your
Baby in a Birth Center

- You are committed to giving birth without pain-relief medications.
- You do not feel relaxed in a medical setting and prefer a nonmedical type of atmosphere.
- You feel more confident in a birth setting surrounded by your family and being cared for by staff (and equipment) that is geared toward supporting a labor experience using coping strategies instead of medical pain-relief strategies.
- You may want to return home as soon as possible after giving birth.

Birth centers are often operated by midwives, or midwives and physicians together. The prospect of giving birth in a birth center is usually most appealing to women who want a birth environment where there will be as few medical interventions (including pain-relief interventions) as possible during labor and birth. The birth center is a good option for women who do not want to have their baby in a hospital but also do not want to give birth at home.

There are some in-hospital birth centers that provide a homey family-centered birth environment; they are attached to the hospital or are located on their campus. The in-hospital birth center is a distinct facility, separate from the hospital's labor and delivery unit. Typically, epidurals are not offered in these centers. Depending on your preferences, this type of environment may also be a perfectly suitable option for you. A birth center within a hospital, however, may not operate in the same way an out-of-hospital birth center does, and its care practices and staffing may be more like hospital care than birth center care.

If you choose to have your baby in a birth center, a certified nurse-midwife (CNM) will most likely be your primary caregiver. Although in birth centers midwives and obstetricians work together, it is the midwife who will likely attend to the birth of your baby, unless the obstetrician is needed due to a complication. Your health care provider must determine that you are a healthy woman with a low-risk pregnancy in order for you to give birth to your baby in a birth center. Birth centers provide care to women throughout their pregnancy, labor and birth, and postpartum period.

The birth center itself is characterized by a homelike atmosphere that is less high tech in appearance than a typical hospital maternity unit. If you are laboring in a birth center and at some point need emergency medical intervention, you will be transferred to a hospital.

Around 15 percent of women who begin their labor in a birth center need to transfer to a hospital. Of these women, only 2 percent transfer due to an emergency. The remainder are transported to the hospital primarily due to slow progress or because the mom requests anesthesia.[5]

Birth centers promote a relaxed, private, nonclinical environment in which a variety of nonmedical pain-management approaches can be accommodated. Birth centers do *not* offer epidurals, and they usually (although not always) do *not* offer narcotic injections. Birth centers are not equipped to perform cesarean section deliveries. In fact, the cesarean section rate for women who began their labor in birth centers is around 4 percent.

ARE WOMEN WHO HAVE THEIR BABIES IN BIRTH CENTERS SATISFIED?

In one study, 98 percent of women who chose to have their babies in a birth center said they would return to give birth in the future, or recommend the birth center to a friend.[6]

At-a-Glance Comparison

*Potential Advantages of Having Your
Baby in the Hospital*

- It's nothing like home. You will have all the equipment
  and staff available in the unlikely event that there is a
  medical emergency with you or your baby.
- Hospitals can manage the high-risk patient or women
  who have medical conditions that may need to be
  monitored and treated.
- There is a variety of medical caregivers to attend to your
  (and your baby's) medical needs.
- Some larger hospitals often have perinatologists (also called
  maternal-fetal specialists) on staff who specialize in the
  care of women who have medically complicated
  pregnancies. If you are considered high risk, these
  specialists may also be involved in your prenatal care.
- Many hospitals have special-care nurseries for newborns
  with health complications or those who need to be
  monitored more closely.
- Many more hospitals now have labor, delivery, recovery, and
  postpartum (LDRP) rooms where you stay from check-in to
  checkout. And still others have labor, delivery, and recovery
  (LDR) rooms that do not require you to move until after
  the baby is born and you have had some time to recover.
- More hospitals are adding complementary and alternative
  pain-relief techniques to use in combination with medical
  pain relief.

*Potential Disadvantages of Having Your
Baby in the Hospital*

- It's nothing like home. You may have to labor in one
  room, but in the unlikely event that there is a medical
  emergency with you or your baby, you may have to move
  to another room to give birth.
- You may have restrictions on who and how many family
  and friends may attend the childbirth.

- Your eating and drinking may be limited in some hospitals.
- Your movement may be restricted if routine IV and monitoring is used (although you may request no IV and no monitoring, if you want to remain mobile for as long as possible).

Potential Advantages of Having Your Baby in a Birth Center

- It's more like home. You will *not* have access to an epidural. If you are committed to avoiding the use of medical pain relief, you may consider this an advantage.
- You will have a private, family-oriented birth setting with fewer restrictions than a hospital *and* fewer unfamiliar hospital staff interacting with you.
- The pain-management approach is based on the use of nonmedical relaxation and coping methods such as position changes, massage, hydrotherapy, and continuous presence of the care provider (see chapter six). The staff working with you is skilled in this type of birth, and the birth center is equipped with a full array of labor and birth support devices (which could include all or many of the following: baths, showers, birth balls, aromatherapy, music).
- There is no use of Pitocin, IVs, or electronic fetal monitors. (The midwife monitors the contractions and fetal heart rate using her touch and a portable device called a Doppler.)
- Midwifery care is provided as your primary care throughout pregnancy and during childbirth.

Potential Disadvantages of Having Your Baby in a Birth Center

- It's more like home. You will *not* have access to an epidural, a disadvantage if you change your mind or your labor is more difficult than you expected. (You can transfer to the hospital if you opt for the epidural.)
- You will not have access to most other forms of medical

pain relief, if nonmedical pain-management measures are not effective for you.

- In the unlikely event that there is an emergency with you or your newborn, you or the baby would need to transfer to a hospital.
- You may not be allowed to stay long after recovery (depending upon your birth center's policy).
- Although birth centers have obstetricians, they may not always be on-site; if a nonurgent medical complication arises that requires attention from a physician, you may have to transfer to a hospital.

WHO *ARE* THESE PEOPLE?

In a survey of over fifteen hundred new moms, 29 percent reported they had never, or had only briefly, met the clinician who attended their birth.[7]

Where you give birth will determine *who* will attend to your needs (and the needs of your newborn) from the moment you arrive on the unit until you are discharged. The caregivers will vary from hospital to hospital. Some of the professionals listed in this chapter are more likely to be found in a hospital setting and others are more likely to be in birth centers.

In both settings the people who will attend to you and your family while you give birth will vary. For example, the caregivers who will be a part of your birth experience in a larger, urban hospital may include some professionals you might not see in a smaller hospital and, conversely, the smaller community hospitals may have professionals and labor support personnel you might not typically find in a larger hospital.

Depending upon where you choose to give birth, the following professionals may be in attendance at one point or another during your labor, birth, and postpartum period:

Your Obstetrician

AVAILABLE IN HOSPITAL: YES
BIRTH CENTER: AT TIMES

An obstetrician (an OB or OB/GYN) is a medical doctor who has received training in normal and high-risk obstetrics and women's health care. Obstetricians are licensed physicians and may be board certified in obstetrics and gynecology. Usually, obstetricians work in hospitals, but they may also deliver babies in birth centers. Most babies born in the United States are delivered by obstetricians.

An obstetrician typically provides your prenatal care throughout your pregnancy, in addition to caring for you during labor and arriving to assist with your baby's birth. In some obstetric practices, during your pregnancy you may be attended to by other clinicians who work in collaboration with the obstetrician, such as nurses, nurse-midwives, and childbirth educators.

You might be surprised to learn that typically, of all those who surround you during labor and birth, your obstetrician is also the person who spends the *least* amount of time with you during labor. In fact, you may already be aware that the obstetrician who attends your birth may be someone you don't know very well, if at all, unless you are lucky enough to go into labor on a day your obstetrician is scheduled to work.

FOR MORE INFORMATION

The American College of Obstetricians and
Gynecologists
409 Twelfth Street, SW
P.O. Box 96920
Washington, D.C. 20090-6920
www.acog.org

Your Labor and Delivery Nurse

AVAILABLE IN HOSPITAL: YES
BIRTH CENTER: AT TIMES

> A labor and delivery nurse (or obstetrical nurse) is a reg-
> istered nurse with a bachelor's or master's degree who has
> specialized in caring for women and newborns during
> labor, birth, and postpartum period.

The labor and delivery nurse is on the front line of care for
laboring women. This nurse may be your most important ally
and is often the first person you will meet once you arrive on
the maternity unit. It is the labor and delivery nurse's goal to establish "rapport, trust, and effective communication" with you
during childbirth.[8] The quality of the support given to you
during labor by your nurse will have a direct impact on your
sense of satisfaction with your childbirth experience.[9]

Your nurse is the person who spends the most time with you,
providing labor support and medical care throughout labor,
childbirth, and the postpartum period. She will get you and your
partner settled into your room, check your vital signs, and make
sure you are comfortable. She will administer your medications
(if you need any), place an IV if one is necessary, and may do
cervical checks (exams) to determine your labor progress. The
labor and delivery nurse provides bedside care and is most likely
the first person who will assess and continue to stay in touch
with your pain-management needs throughout labor and birth.

Your labor and delivery nurse will work in partnership with
your obstetrician and anesthesiologist, keeping them aware of your
(and your baby's) status, and communicating with them about
your labor progress and comfort level. She also acts as your labor
support person, especially if you do not have a doula or midwife
present. Your labor and delivery nurse will be present when you
deliver, even if you are also attended by a midwife or doula.

Patient education is a big part of your labor and delivery nurse's role while you are in the hospital. If you are a first-time mom, you will often learn things you didn't even think about before arriving on the maternity unit. The labor and delivery nurse will, of course, keep you aware of what is happening to your body, and your baby, throughout labor and birth. She will teach you how to properly care for yourself during recovery, show you how to properly breast-feed, and demonstrate how to bathe and care for your baby. From cradle cap to umbilical cord care, your labor and delivery nurse will cover it all by the time you are ready to go home.

FOR MORE INFORMATION

The Association of Women's Health, Obstetric and
Neonatal Nurses
2000 L Street, Suite 740
Washington, D.C. 20036
www.awhonn.org

Your Anesthesiologist

AVAILABLE IN HOSPITAL: YES
BIRTH CENTER: NO

An anesthesiologist is a medical doctor who has completed specialized training in the field of anesthesiology. The anesthesiologist in the maternity unit manages the care of both the mother and the baby. Some (typically larger) hospitals have anesthesiologists who specialize in obstetrics, known as obstetric anesthesiologists. These physicians work closely with the obstetricians, midwives, and labor and delivery nurses to assess and manage your pain.

Most likely you will not know the anesthesiologist who attends to you on the labor and delivery unit. If during labor you request an epidural, your anesthesiologist will meet with you, take a brief medical history, and ask you to determine your own pain level, typically using a scale that asks you to rate your pain level from one to ten.

Your anesthesiologist will collaborate with your obstetrician and nurse (see page 80, "When Can You Get an Epidural?"), and your nurse will assist your anesthesiologist with the placement of the epidural. The anesthesiologist and your labor and delivery nurse (or midwife, if you have one) will work together to assess your pain level throughout the rest of your labor, birth, and postpartum period.

The availability of anesthesiologists varies from hospital to hospital. And, even within the same hospital, the anesthesiologists available to the maternity patients (and other patients) can vary, depending upon the time of day, how busy the maternity unit is, or how many anesthesiologists are on duty at once. Smaller hospitals may not have an anesthesiologist who works in-house (in the hospital) twenty-four hours a day, seven days a week. It is important to know how the anesthesia coverage works in the hospital where you plan to have your baby. If you go into labor in the middle of the night and the anesthesiologist does not report to work until the next morning, your plans for pain relief may be delayed.

In larger hospitals and busier maternity units, anesthesiologists are typically on the unit or available to the maternity unit around the clock. This does not guarantee that there will be no delays, but it does improve the likelihood that you will be attended to by an anesthesiologist promptly, should you decide you need an epidural or other pain medication.

FOR MORE INFORMATION

The Society for Obstetric Anesthesia and Perinatology
2 Summit Park Drive, Suite 140

Cleveland, OH 44131-2571
www.soap.org

The American Society of Anesthesiologists
520 N. Northwest Highway
Park Ridge, IL 60068-2573
www.asahq.org

An additional resource:
www.painfreebirthing.com

Your Nurse-Anesthetist

AVAILABLE IN HOSPITAL: YES
BIRTH CENTER: NO

A nurse-anesthetist is a registered nurse who has a degree
from an accredited nurse-anesthesia program. The nurse-
anesthetist works closely with the obstetrician, midwife,
and labor and delivery nurse to assess and manage your pain.

In some hospitals, your anesthesia may be provided by a
nurse-anesthetist, either working alone or in partnership with
an anesthesiologist. A nurse-anesthetist, also called a CRNA, or
certified registered nurse-anesthetist, is a nurse with specialized
training in the administration and management of anesthesia.
CRNAs provide anesthesia in approximately two-thirds of all
rural hospitals in the United States.

FOR MORE INFORMATION

The American Association of Nurse Anesthetists
222 S. Prospect Avenue
Park Ridge, IL 60068
www.aana.com

Your Certified Nurse-Midwife

AVAILABLE IN HOSPITAL: YES (SOME)
BIRTH CENTER: YES

Approximately 10 percent of babies born in the United States are delivered by a certified nurse-midwife. A certified nurse-midwife (CNM) has a degree in nursing and a degree in nurse-midwifery, and has passed the American College of Nurse-Midwives board examination to obtain certification.

Midwives typically care for women who are considered to have a low-risk pregnancy and who anticipate a low-risk birth. Although nurse-midwives are medically trained, with a nursing background, they are often oriented toward a nonmedical birth approach and many employ a variety of complementary and alternative methods of pain management. Certified nurse-midwives may practice in birth centers or hospitals, or at home births. Some hospitals have midwives on staff as a part of their obstetric practice, and the obstetricians and midwives collaboratively provide care for their patients.

The role of the midwife is to provide you with emotional support and patient education, in addition to handling all aspects of your prenatal care and providing continuous labor support during childbirth. Midwives provide postpartum care as well. Midwives perform many of the tasks of an obstetrician: they prescribe medications, attend to the birth of the baby, and suture the mother if needed. Midwives do *not* perform cesarean deliveries, however, and if one is needed, you will be referred to an obstetrician. If this occurs, your midwife may remain with you to provide support and continuity of care during the procedure.

FOR MORE INFORMATION

The American College of Nurse-Midwives
8403 Colesville Road, Suite 1550
Silver Spring, MD 20910-6374
www.acnm.org.

In addition to certified nurse-midwives, there are other types of
midwives who may be available in your area such as:

Your Certified Professional Midwife

AVAILABLE IN HOSPITAL: RARELY
BIRTH CENTER: YES

A certified professional midwife is a title for midwives
who have met certification standards established by the North
American Registry of Midwives (NARM), but who do not
also have a nursing degree. These midwives typically attend
births within birth centers (or homes), and far less often in
hospitals.

FOR MORE INFORMATION

The North American Registry of Midwives
5257 Rosestone Drive
Lilburn, GA 30047
www.narm.org

To learn more about midwives, including other types of midwives not described here:

Midwives Alliance of North America
375 Rockbridge Road
Suite 172-313
Lilburn, GA 30047
www.mana.org

Your Family Physician

AVAILABLE IN HOSPITAL: YES
BIRTH CENTER: YES

> In some locales, particularly in rural areas, family physicians, not obstetricians, may provide obstetrical care for birthing mothers. The family physician is a medical doctor who is a specialist in family practice and is typically responsible for the health of the entire family, not just the mom-to-be.

In parts of the country where obstetricians are not as prevalent, family physicians are more likely to provide care to pregnant women and attend their childbirth.

FOR MORE INFORMATION

American Academy of Family Physicians
11400 Tomahawk Creek Parkway
Leawood, KS 66211-2672
www.aafp.org

Your Doula

AVAILABLE IN HOSPITAL: YES
BIRTH CENTER: YES

> A birth doula is a birth assistant who is trained and experienced in labor support and childbirth. To become certified by DONA [Doulas of North America] International, doulas have a minimum of twenty-eight hours of labor support training, read several required books, must attend

three births in which they are evaluated in writing by the doctor and nurse, or midwife and the mother. The number of doula-attended births has grown dramatically in the last decade and some hospitals are now offering doula services for their maternity patients.

The role of the birth doula is to provide continuous emotional, physical, and informational support to the laboring woman and her partner throughout labor and childbirth. According to Penny Simkin, one of the founders of DONA International, "The doula's goal is to help the woman have a safe and satisfying birth experience as the woman defines it."

You and your doula have the advantage of knowing each other before you get to the labor and delivery room, whereas you are unlikely to know your nurse or possibly the doctor who will deliver your baby. Often the doula will meet with you a few times before your due date to get to know you and your partner and discuss your childbirth and pain-relief preferences. The doula may help you draw up your birth plan (see page 272), provide you with educational materials, and then join you at home or meet you at the hospital or birth center once your labor begins. The doula provides continuous attention and support to the laboring mother in a unique way. Unlike your labor and delivery nurse, she does not have other patients to attend to and does not leave your side. Your doula (unlike some partners) will not feel overwhelmed or anxious seeing you in labor. She has expertise in being with and providing support to women who are in labor and she will know what you need and how to meet your needs in a calm, knowing, and supportive manner.

TRY AN "EPI-DOULA"

Some may think doulas are primarily for women who prefer to use little or no pain medication. While a few doulas attend only these types of births, most doulas will support you in your decision to have the type of birth you want. Even if you receive an epidural and you are entirely pain-free, you and your partner can still benefit from the encouragement, comfort, and practical assistance offered by the continued presence of a doula.

A doula is not a clinician. Although a few doulas are also trained as nurses, most typically have no medical training and will not provide you with medical advice or medical care. Doulas do not deliver babies.

The doula's constant support while you labor does not replace your partner's; in fact, she supports you both throughout your labor. In a long labor, the doula's presence means your partner is able to rest and take a break. The doula can offer assistance and ideas for your partner on how to best meet your emotional and physical needs as your labor progresses. She will help you remember and implement the breathing and relaxation techniques you may have learned, and she may provide you with massage and touch to enhance your relaxation and attempt to reduce your discomfort. A doula provides verbal reassurance and encouragement and will help you with your positioning and movement to keep your labor progressing and to attempt to keep you as comfortable as possible.

FOR MORE INFORMATION

DONA International
P.O. Box 626
Jasper, IN 47547
www.dona.org

Childbirth and Postpartum Professional Association
P.O. Box 491448
Lawrenceville, GA 30049
www.cappa.net

The Association of Labor Assistants and Childbirth
Educators (ALACE)
P.O. Box 390436
Cambridge, MA 02139
www.alace.org

The National Association of Childbearing Centers
3123 Gottschall Road
Perkiomenville, PA 18074
www.birthcenters.org

Two

YOUR LABOR PAIN—
HOW PAINFUL IS IT?
REALLY.

We had dinner recently with some friends who told us about their experience checking into the labor and delivery suite at a renowned teaching hospital for the birth of their first daughter. After completing their admitting paperwork, our friend Tracy and her husband, John, followed their nurse down the hall to their room on the labor and delivery unit. They were startled by the sounds throughout the hallway of women moaning loudly in labor. Tracy, who described to us her increasing anxiety as they approached her room, finally stopped to ask the nurse, "Am I going to be in that much pain?" The nurse assured her with the standard explanation: "Labor pain is different for every woman," and got them settled comfortably into their room. We all laughed with familiar recognition at the predictable punch line, when John told us that six hours later, the sounds coming from Tracy's room were louder than those they had heard earlier that evening on their naive journey down the hall.

Labor pain should not remain a mystery until you arrive on the labor and delivery unit. There is enough historical, medical, and anecdotal information, based on women's own personal experiences, to prepare for what to expect during your labor and delivery.

In this chapter you will learn:

- Why it is important to know what to expect.
- How labor pain has been described by women using pain-measurement scales.
- How some women make a distinction between *pain* and *suffering* during childbirth.
- Key factors that can impact the intensity of your labor pain.
- How physicians, nurses, midwives, childbirth educators, and doulas describe the pain of childbirth and what they recommend you do to prepare for a positive birth experience.

How Painful Is it?

DID YOU KNOW? *The American College of Obstetricians and Gynecologists (ACOG) released the following statement regarding labor pain: "Labor results in severe pain for many women. There is no other circumstance where it is considered acceptable for a person to experience untreated severe pain, amenable to safe intervention, while under a physician's care. In the absence of a medical contraindication, maternal request is a sufficient medical indication for pain relief during labor. Pain management should be provided whenever medically indicated."*[1]

Most women report that childbirth rates as one of the most physically intense and challenging experiences in their lives. There is no specific medical definition or one-size-fits-all description of labor pain, and several factors are thought to influence the severity and duration of pain experienced during labor and delivery.

DID YOU KNOW? *"Popular books written for pregnant women often understate the degree of pain experienced during birth, and may overstate the effectiveness of childbirth preparation in reducing pain."*—*Marci Lobel, Ph.D., associate professor of psychology and director of the Stony Brook Pregnancy Project at Stony Brook University, an expert on pregnancy and mental health.*

Two major childbirth magazines, one American, the other British, recently conducted surveys that polled their readers' perceptions about their own childbirth experiences. All of the women who participated had recently given birth; both surveys showed that most women are *not* prepared for the intensity of pain involved in labor and delivery. Many women who were surveyed voiced dissatisfaction with the fact that the reality of the physical challenges of childbirth was downplayed or glossed over by their caregivers, childbirth educators, or others. In the survey done by *American Baby* magazine, the vast majority of women who responded "found labor extremely painful."[2]

The reality of labor should not be downplayed in an attempt to prevent you from feeling anxious. Chances are you already feel apprehensive about what to expect in the delivery room, whether this is your first baby or not. When others describe childbirth in terms that are meant to soften the severity, intensity, and duration of labor, you are put at a disadvantage. If you are unable to realistically anticipate the sensations you may experience during childbirth, including pain, you may find the experience overwhelming and feel unprepared to make clear, well-informed decisions regarding the types of coping strategies and pain-relief options you may prefer to use once labor pain begins.

Advice given in the form of clichés, although often well meaning, can mask the reality of labor and dismiss your fears as invalid and unimportant. Often women hear, "The pain you will feel is good pain," or "It will all be worthwhile," or "You will forget about the pain." These statements do nothing to address your fear and anxiety, and instead minimize the importance of dealing with the difficult emotions you may be feeling.

Not all women, in the full intensity of labor, are able to (or wish to) view the pain they experience as "good pain" by reframing it as a positive part of their childbirth experience. You will almost certainly feel that it was all worthwhile once you begin bonding with your newborn. However, this conclusion implies that severe pain is a necessary part of giving birth, and does little to ease the fears of women who want to make every effort to avoid pain and suffering during labor.

Finally, telling a pregnant woman who is anxious about her impending labor and birth that she will forget about the pain is insensitive and untrue. It is a statement that does not provide comfort or extend empathy during a time when both are needed. Unless you are given a specific medication that provides amnesia-like effects, it is unlikely that you will ever forget your memories of childbirth. In fact, studies have shown that women's memories of giving birth are recorded accurately for decades and last a lifetime.[3]

Rather than dismissing your fear of labor pain with platitudes, your caregivers, family members, friends, and partners should strive to encourage your full awareness of what to expect in the labor and delivery room and promote an understanding and acceptance of the many safe and effective pain-management options you may wish to choose.

A Brief Description of the Stages of Labor

Medical experts divide labor into three stages. The amount of time spent in each stage varies among women. Most women will go to their hospital or birth center at the beginning of the first stage of labor or right after their water breaks. You and your obstetrician or midwife will need to determine when it is appropriate for you to arrive at your birth setting.

> **Did You Know?** *When labor first begins, if you start feeling uncomfortable, you can use a variety of pain-management strategies at home, such as walking, taking a warm shower, having your partner massage you, or just relaxing with an activity you enjoy.*

The first stage of labor refers to the time from the beginning of labor up to the point of full cervical dilation, which is ten centimeters. This is almost always the longest part of a woman's labor and can last from a few hours to longer than eighteen hours in some women. This first stage of labor itself is divided into two distinct subphases known as the *latent* and *active* phases. The latent phase refers to the beginning of cervical dilation to approximately three to four centimeters and typically progresses more slowly than the next phases of labor. The active phase describes a faster rate of cervical dilation and begins when the cervix has dilated to approximately three to four centimeters and ends when the cervix has fully dilated to ten centimeters.

A transition period occurs at the end of the first stage of labor. During this time your contractions may become more intense, closer together, and (if you are without pain relief) more painful. Transition can last from a few minutes up to a few hours. Some women experience shaking, shivering, and nausea during the transition period. A very normal and common response many women experience during this part of labor is feeling out of control or thinking it is impossible to continue. During this phase women often feel physically and emotionally drained. Good labor support is vital during this period, especially for women who have opted for no medical pain relief.

The second stage refers to the time between full cervical dilation (ten centimeters) and the birth of the infant. This is the phase during which women become even more active in the birth process by pushing the baby through the birth canal. This stage can last from a few minutes to as long as several hours, and is generally shorter for repeat moms. Some women report a sense of relief of pain during this phase as they finally give birth to the baby; others find the pressure and stretching as the baby exits to be more painful. The exact sensations experienced as the baby descends will vary from woman to woman and are impacted by the type of pain relief you have chosen.

The third stage refers to the time from delivery of the infant to delivery of the placenta. It is typically the shortest part of a woman's labor and usually lasts less than ten minutes, but may last up to thirty minutes. This final stage of labor, for most women (who do not have an effective pain-relief method), marks the end of their intense pain or discomfort; the placenta is usually expelled without much pain or effort.

WHAT EXACTLY IS LABOR PAIN? AND WHAT DOES IT FEEL LIKE?

There is no one precise answer to these questions. In fact, no one knows exactly why labor hurts; medical, scientific, and religious communities have debated this topic for thousands of years. Labor pain is a unique type of pain, since it is not associated with injury or disease but is the result of a normal, healthy bodily process: childbirth. The perception of labor pain is thought to include more than just the physical sensations of your uterine contractions followed by your baby's birth. It is thought that the human experience of any type of pain, including labor pain, may be influenced by a variety of factors including your age, life experiences, cultural and gender expectations, and possibly previous trauma or painful past experiences. The pain associated with childbirth is different from other types of physical pain since it is time limited and characterized by a beginning, middle, and end. Labor pain typically does not start all at once; for most women it is gradual and begins with a mild to moderate amount of pain, which over the course of several hours increases in intensity.

The initial sensation of labor pain is a result of uterine contractions and may be felt not just in the abdomen but in the lower back, the sacrum (the pelvis), and the upper thighs. Typically the pain associated with contractions begins as a dull cramping sensation. When the contractions intensify in strength, so does the laboring woman's pain level. Most often, there is a break from the pain in between contractions. This allows you to rest for a period before managing the next contraction. First-time mothers typically experience more pain during the early stage of labor, whereas repeat moms report more intense pain toward the end of the first stage and in the second stage of their labor. This increase in pain during late labor, for repeat moms, is due to the baby descending more quickly through the birth canal than in first-time moms.[4]

As labor progresses, during the pushing stage, the vaginal walls stretch and the baby pushes down on the perineum (the area between the vagina and rectum). The mother is not just pushing because her caregivers prompt her to; she is experiencing an intense *urge* to push at this time. Many women describe the pain sensation at this point, as the baby descends, as more of a sharp, stinging sensation. This distinct sensation is often referred to as the "ring of fire." Not all women experience this, and certainly most women who have received numbing medications or an epidural do not feel pain as the baby exits. Some women report experiencing pain during the repair of the vaginal opening if an episiotomy is performed (an episiotomy is a controversial procedure that involves the surgical cutting of the vaginal opening to attempt to minimize tearing as the baby exits the birth canal). If, however, numbing medication has been given, or women are using an epidural, any repair stitching of tissue or muscle will not be painful.

WHAT EXACTLY IS BACK LABOR AND IS IT REALLY MORE PAINFUL?

You may have heard women describe their labor pain as back labor. Women who have back labor feel the discomfort and pain of their contractions primarily in their lower back rather than in their abdominal area. Often, but not always, back labor is a result of the baby being in the posterior fetal position, meaning that the baby is facing up toward the mom's front rather than in the proper birthing position, facing downward toward the mom's tailbone.

Back labor is often described as more intense than abdominal labor because, unlike most abdominal labor pains, it is often characterized by steady pressure and pain, with no break or rest period in between contractions. Some women feel only back pain, with no abdominal discomfort; others feel most of their labor in their lower back and hip area, with some abdominal pain. Back labor can be relieved by the same measures used for abdominal labor, but other methods may help ease the pain associated with this particular type of labor. These include position changes, laboring while in a hands-and-knees position, and applying pressure massage or warm and cold compresses to the lower back.

WHAT CAUSES LABOR TO BEGIN?

Contrary to what you may have heard, as far as we know, labor is not brought on by your favorite Mexican food or a large pizza with "the works." In fact, exactly what causes labor to begin is unknown; even today, the whole process is regarded as complex and poorly understood. Changes in the uterus or hormones produced by the mother or infant may activate the start of labor. Today's theories on this topic suggest that there are signals from the baby (I'm ready to come out), from the mother (I'm ready to get rid of this passenger), or from the placenta (I've done my job). These signals could be metabolic, hormonal, chronologic, or some combination of all three. Making the matter more complex is the problem of why some women go into labor prematurely (before thirty-seven weeks), and it is likely that whatever triggers preterm labor is different from what triggers full-term labor.[5]

THE PAIN MEASUREMENT SCALES

DID YOU KNOW? *Only 1 percent of women report experiencing no pain during childbirth.*[6]

Several studies have actually measured the amount of pain women feel during labor, with the goal of defining, as precisely as possible, the intensity of pain women experience throughout labor. The purpose of measuring labor pain is to gain information that can help in the development of effective labor pain–relief interventions and, as important, to contribute to educating women as they prepare for their own childbirth experience.

The most widely used pain-measurement scale is the McGill Pain Questionnaire (MPQ), which has been used throughout many countries, including the United States, to assess the nature and intensity of labor pain. The questionnaire uses words that are commonly used by physicians and patients in their descriptions of pain.

The MPQ is given to women during labor. Women in

labor are asked to respond to the descriptive words used as pain indicators. The words are read out loud to the women at the start of labor and throughout labor and delivery. The women then choose one word from each category that best reflects what they are experiencing at that time. In some studies they are also asked to recall the pain of their labor twenty-four to forty-eight hours after giving birth.

The following results were shown in the overall pain ratings during labor, using the MPQ in a number of different studies[7]:

	First-time moms	Repeat moms
Rated mild to moderate pain	9%	24%
Rated severe pain	30%	30%
Rated very severe pain	38%	35%
Rated horrible or excruciating pain	23%	11%

The MPQ has found that labor is severe for most women. But keep reading. You will learn how to manage, reduce, or eliminate these painful sensations.

HOW WOMEN FEEL DURING LABOR—*EMOTIONALLY*

You've just read descriptions of *what* women felt during childbirth, but it may surprise you to learn *how* women felt during childbirth. A national survey, called *Listening to Mothers,* was recently conducted for the Maternity Center Association. The survey, which polled over fifteen hundred women within twenty-four months of giving birth, was the first ever in the

United States to ask women directly about their childbirth experiences.[8] The results of the survey revealed that women experience a number of different and sometimes seemingly opposing emotions while giving birth. These women were asked to choose, from a list of randomly ordered positive and negative descriptive words, the ones that best described how they felt during labor. The word selection was as follows:

Positive: *Alert, Capable, Confident, Calm, Unafraid,*
   Powerful
Negative: *Overwhelmed, Weak, Frightened, Agitated,*
   Groggy, Helpless

The results indicate that many women experience conflicting emotions during childbirth. It is encouraging to see that most women chose words that described *positive* feelings during labor. Most of the women chose the words *alert* (82 percent), *capable* (77 percent), *confident* (65 percent), and *calm* (63 percent); fewer described their feelings as *unafraid* (44 percent) and *powerful* (34 percent).

Many also chose the negative words *overwhelmed* (48 percent), *weak* (41 percent), *frightened* (39 percent), and *helpless* (25 percent) to describe how they felt during labor and delivery. Some mothers described an unusual combination of emotions indicating that they felt both *confident* and *overwhelmed* (24 percent), *agitated* and *calm* (15 percent), *groggy* and *alert* (14 percent), and *powerful* and *weak* (7 percent). The survey showed that repeat moms were much more likely than first-time moms to choose positive words to describe their feelings toward childbirth. For more information on this survey, go to www.maternitywise.org.

The physical experience of labor is known to be unique to each individual woman. This description can also be applied to the emotional aspects of childbirth. Women typically feel a variety of emotions throughout their childbirth experiences and of course can feel more than one emotion at a time. For instance, it is not surprising that a woman could feel both confident in her ability to give birth and overwhelmed by the physical experience of labor. Childbirth, regardless of one's choice of pain management, is a highly emotional event and an extraordinary physical challenge, during which most women feel a number of different emotions.

Is There a Difference Between Pain and Suffering?
The vast majority of women want pain relief and do not make a distinction between the experience of pain and the experience of suffering. For most women, the pain itself causes suffering. Some women, however, believe there is a meaningful difference between *feeling* the pain of childbirth and *suffering* from the pain of childbirth. For these women, the experience of pain is not necessarily objectionable. Can pain exist *without* suffering during childbirth? There is not a "right" answer to this question. The matter is quite complex, and very much depends on each individual woman's values and perspectives.

Why Do Some Women Choose to Embrace the Pain of Childbirth?
Some women who choose not to use pain-relief medications believe that the presence of pain, or specifically their ability to meet the challenge of coping with their pain, plays an important role in contributing to their sense of satisfaction with the overall birth experience.

Birth philosophies that promote this approach suggest that with proper preparation and good labor support, women who give birth in their preferred birth environment without modern pain relief can have a rewarding and positive birth experience.

Women who choose to give birth in this manner often speak of their sense of reward, empowerment, and spiritual fulfillment after giving birth without the use of pain-relief medications or other medical interventions. You will read some of these women's comments and birth stories in chapters six and ten.

Most women who use pain relief in the form of narcotics and epidurals do not view their pain as adding value to their birth experience. In fact, many women report that the pain itself detracted from their ability to experience the joy and fulfillment they wished to experience during childbirth. Once adequate pain relief was achieved, they were able to feel the joy and emotional charge connected with giving birth.

Even women who are emotionally and physically prepared for childbirth, feel confident in their ability to give birth, have excellent labor support, and are in their preferred birth environment may suffer with their labor pain and wish to use pain relief. These women do not view the birth experience as a challenge they either want to or must meet without the benefit of pain relief, and they are willing to tolerate the potential risks, side effects, and interventions necessary to have a more comfortable labor and birth. You will read some of these women's comments and birth stories in chapters four and ten.

THE MOST COMMON FACTORS THAT CAN IMPACT YOUR LABOR PAIN

DID YOU KNOW? *"In an analysis of factors thought to influence labor pain, which included fear of pain, confidence, concern about the outcome of labor, frequency of contractions, menstrual pain, and size (weight) of the baby,* confidence *consistently emerged as the most significant predictor of first stage labor pain."*—Nancy Lowe, Ph.D., certified nurse-midwife[9]

There are many complex variables that impact how much pain is experienced during childbirth. The experience of labor is different for every woman, and the same woman can have a very different labor with each childbirth. The factors that influence labor pain are generally thought to be a combination of physical, emotional, cultural, and psychological responses to childbirth.

In this section we list the most common factors thought to

influence the amount of pain you may experience during labor; some you will have control over, some you will not.

1. **Your own sense of confidence:** Women's confidence toward their own successful use of pain-management strategies during childbirth has been shown to predict lower levels of pain during the beginning stage of labor (less than three centimeters dilated) but not during active labor (four to seven centimeters dilated).[10] Confidence has also been associated with influencing women's perceptions of childbirth as a positive or negative experience. Women who approach labor and delivery with a feeling of confidence in their own ability to manage or cope with their pain are more likely to report feeling that their birth experience was a positive one. Confidence in the belief that your pain-relief requests will be met appropriately by caregivers is also an important consideration in the overall childbirth experience.

2. **The birthing environment:** Giving birth in the environment that suits your overall birth plan and reflects your expectations for the type of childbirth you want, including your pain-relief preferences, can directly determine the amount of pain you may experience during labor. If you know you want an epidural, you may want to give birth in a hospital with twenty-four-hour anesthesiology availability. Women who prefer to manage most or all of their labor with "low-tech" pain-relief interventions, such as birth balls (see page 197), water immersion, and massage, may be best served in a hospital that has a maternity unit where these resources are available, or in a birth center that provides more of these options than in a traditional hospital setting.

3. **First baby or repeat:** The number of births you have had can impact the intensity of your labor pain. First-time moms rate labor pain as worse than expected in all

three stages of labor. Repeat moms rate labor as less
severe than expected in stage one of labor, but describe
stage two of labor as more painful than they expected.[11]
It has been suggested that for repeat moms, this increase
in pain during the later stage of labor may be due to the
fact that the muscles used in birth have become more
supple and "experienced" from previous pregnancies
and, as a result, the baby may descend very quickly,
causing more intense pain than in previous birth(s).

4. **Dystocia,** literally, "difficult childbirth": Dystocia is
diagnosed when cervical dilation does not progress
while contractions are still taking place, and the baby
does not descend through the birth canal. In other
words, with dystocia, the mother is still having contractions, but she does not continue to dilate normally and her labor is obstructed. Dystocia is one of
the most common reasons for cesarean delivery in the
United States.[12] It is thought to be associated with more
intense labor pain.

5. **Family and social support:** Your family, partner,
close friend, doula, or midwife who provides continuous support during labor can strongly influence
how you cope with pain. Family and social support
during labor and birth may not actually reduce your
pain level, but the praise, encouragement, and
emotional support of others can help you have a more
positive overall birth experience (see the section "Labor
Support," page 180, in chapter six).

6. **History of dysmenorrhea (menstrual cramps):**
Some studies have suggested a link between labor-pain
intensity and a woman's history of severe menstrual
cramps.[13] It is thought that women who suffer from
severe menstrual cramps produce more pain-causing
blood chemicals known as prostaglandins. These
prostaglandins produce more-intense contractions, a
condition common to both severe menstrual pain and
intense labor pain.

7. **Oxytocin (or Pitocin):** Oxytocin is a drug given to laboring women to speed up labor. Oxytocin increases the strength and frequency of your contractions. This increase often causes a rise in the intensity of labor pain. It has been suggested that the epidural increases the need for women to receive oxytocin during labor, but few studies compare the timing of epidurals with the actual initiation of oxytocin. Research suggests that the oxytocin itself produces a more intense and painful labor, which then increases women's requests for epidural pain relief.[14]

8. **Size of baby:** A large baby is considered a baby with an estimated weight in utero of eight pounds, thirteen ounces or more (the medical term used to describe these biggie-sized infants is *macrosomia*). A large baby may place more stress on the mom's body during its descent through the birth canal. It is thought that the compatibility between the size of the baby and the mom's birth passage may have a direct impact on the intensity of labor pain. If the baby is large but the mother's body can accommodate its size fairly well, then she may not experience any additional pain or discomfort. If the mom is small and the baby is large, however, there is likely to be more stress on her perineal area as the baby makes its exit.

9. **Maternal position:** The position of women during labor and delivery has been a controversial issue in maternity care for some time. In the United States, birthing women are commonly placed in the horizontal position to labor and birth, rather than an upright or squatting position. This preference for birthing in the horizontal position has often been attributed to ensuring the convenience of the physician rather than to enhance the birth process or promote patient comfort.

    It has been demonstrated that women in the sitting or standing position during early labor report lower pain scores than when they are lying horizontal.[15] However, it is also possible that the position of sitting or standing is not the cause of the pain relief, but rather that women who are able to sit and stand are actually *experiencing less pain* than women whose labor is more intense. Greater labor pain renders some women unable to get up and move around. In general, women find different positions to be more or less comfortable than others, and throughout labor and birth each woman should go with what works best for her.

10. **"Sunny-side up" baby:** Many women suffer from back pain during labor. This pain is often attributed to a baby being in the posterior fetal position, also known as sunny-side up. This is where the baby's face is positioned toward the mom's front, rather than the more common position of the baby facing down, toward the mom's tailbone. However, many women whose babies are in the proper birthing position also report painful back labor.

11. **Caregivers' response to your pain:** Your caregivers' response can help alleviate your pain in various ways. If your caregivers are responding to your cues and following your lead, whenever possible, regarding the type and timing of the pain relief you request, your pain is likely to be diminished. If your caregivers effectively assist you with the use of your preferred coping strategies, they may help minimize your pain throughout your labor or, if you choose medications or an epidural, they may make all the difference by providing you with good support until these medications can be administered. Conversely, if your caregivers' perceptions of your pain intensity differ from your own actual pain experience, you may not receive adequate or timely relief (see chapter eleven for more information on the role of caregivers and your pain relief during childbirth).

12. **Cultural norms:** The perception and expression of labor pain is influenced by women's cultural norms and expectations. During childbirth there is no difference in the pain-intensity ratings among various cultures and ethnic groups.[16] However, women's *response* to pain during childbirth varies greatly among cultures. Each culture influences how women deal with labor pain by defining what is considered appropriate behavior for the expression of their pain. Some cultures dictate that women remain stoic and quiet during birth; other cultures encourage vocalization and free expression of pain.

    An interesting complication to this connection between cultural influences and the management of pain is the suggestion that the cultural norms of the *caregivers* themselves may also influence how a woman's pain is responded to during labor. Some research has suggested that the greater the difference in cultural identity between patient and caregiver, the more likely the caregiver is to interpret the patient's experience of pain inaccurately.[17]

13. **Childbirth education classes:** Research differs on whether childbirth education classes ultimately help women reduce their pain during labor by implementing the relaxation, breathing, and focusing techniques learned in these courses. The success and effectiveness of childbirth preparation courses depend upon a number of factors, including the effectiveness of the person teaching the course, the usefulness of the material covered during the course, and how receptive the pregnant woman is to the approach and techniques used during childbirth preparation training.

    Some research has suggested that the impact of childbirth preparation classes on labor pain is small, and most women who attend these classes may still experience severe pain during labor if they do not receive pain relief or use an effective pain-control technique.[18] Even if there is not a direct connection between your attendance of childbirth preparation courses and the reduction of your labor pain, it may still be of value for you to attend these sessions to learn about the birth process itself and gain an understanding of the hospital's (or birth center's) practices and policies, to ensure that they are in sync with your own preferences and birth philosophy.

ARE YOU PREPARED?: PHYSICIANS, MIDWIVES, LABOR AND DELIVERY NURSES, CHILDBIRTH EDUCATORS, AND DOULAS ANSWER THIS QUESTION AND DESCRIBE LABOR PAIN

Many of the clinicians and caregivers we interviewed reported that women are often unprepared for the amount of pain they experience during childbirth. There is not always agreement on why this is so, but we consistently found that those who work professionally with women in labor and delivery report that women need more accurate information before they reach the delivery room. We asked the following questions of physicians, midwives, labor and delivery nurses, childbirth educators, and doulas, then asked each to give words of advice to help prepare women for their upcoming birth:

1. In general, do you find that women are prepared for the pain involved in childbirth? If yes, to what do you attribute their preparedness? If no, to what do you attribute their lack of preparation?
2. In your practice, how do you typically describe the pain of labor to first-time moms?
3. What advice can you offer to help women feel prepared for childbirth?

This Is What Nurses and Midwives Told Us

Ms. Debbie Pickens, R.N., associate unit manager for labor and delivery, Parkland Memorial Hospital, Dallas, Texas

"No, women are not prepared for the intensity of pain during labor. Even women who have given birth before often forget the intensity of the pain until it hits them again when labor begins. Many women feel they have a higher pain tolerance than they actually do, and very often they underestimate the pain involved in labor.

"It will be like no pain you have ever felt before. The contractions will feel like tightening and cramping, and these sensations will intensify as your labor progresses. The pain will become more forceful and more severe after your water breaks."

Advice to Moms

Ms. Pickens reminds women about the availability of pain-relief options during early labor in an attempt to prepare women ahead of time, before the pain gets too intense, and often reminds her laboring mothers, "You can change your mind at any time and ask for pain relief."

Ms. Lisa Walsh, R.N., a certified nurse-midwife for Women's Health Care and Anna Jaques Hospital, Newburyport, Massachusetts

"I would say most women are not prepared for the pain. However, many young women sail right through and have relatively short labors. They will often be up and around and talking about a second baby. I have wondered if that is because we were meant to have babies in the late teens and early twenties, as we did two hundred years ago. I am usually reassured if women express concern for how they will cope with the pain, versus saying they expect that it won't be bad . . . it may be a more realistic approach, expecting that it will be painful."

Ms. Walsh said she does not describe the pain of childbirth to women. "First of all, because I have no idea how it feels, it kind of makes me feel like an imposter, being a midwife who has never had a baby! I guess I would say that it looks like it hurts like hell, but I don't want to scare them!"

Advice to Moms

"My usual conversation involves encouraging women to keep an open mind and not make any declarations about what they want or how they expect they will manage labor before they have the first few contractions. I encourage women to attend their childbirth classes, to learn about what is normal for labor. By understanding the basic physiology and natural course of events, women may be less frightened by the unknown, and less fear may result in less pain during labor."

Marcia Patterson, a labor and delivery nurse and the unit director of OB Services, Rush Presbyterian St. Luke's Medical Center, Chicago, Illinois

Ms. Patterson, who has over thirty years' experience in obstetric care, told us, "Young women don't prepare themselves for labor pain because they intend to use epidurals. They often don't anticipate having any pain. Women have shortchanged themselves by thinking they can have an epidural without attempting other pain-relief measures. There are several pain-relief alternatives, but many women do not have the confidence or support from their caregivers to access them."

She describes labor pain by asking women, "Did you ever have really bad menstrual cramps? It is like that, except it is intermittent, and as labor progresses they get stronger. It's hard to describe labor, and in particular it is hard to describe the sensations women often feel in the second stage of labor. I sometimes try to describe this part of labor by telling women it feels like you are pushing out a bowling ball. That might sound too graphic, but it is a good comparison!"

Advice to Moms

"I recommend that, before they arrive on the labor and delivery unit, all mothers-to-be learn as much as they can about the process of labor and what to expect once they are admitted to the hospital. Classes are especially helpful because they provide opportunities for interaction with other prospective parents and with the instructor. Discuss with your physician or midwife, during office visits, any special requests or expectations you may have, so that any conflicts can be resolved before your labor begins. Finally, know that you, as a woman, have within yourself the power and resources to labor and give birth."

Ms. Diedre A. Dibal, a certified nurse-midwife at Bethany Women's Care, Kansas City, Kansas

Ms. Dibal describes herself as "a hospital midwife, wife, mother, grandmother, moderate feminist, Catholic, liberal Southern Democrat, and an advocate for my patients!" She told us, "It is impossible for first-time birthers to anticipate the amount of pain involved with labors. There is no way to describe it. The unfortunate part of the token childbirth preparation that most courses offer is that they mislead women into thinking if they breathe in some peculiar pattern while lying flat on their back, tied to a hospital bed with a monitor and an IV in their arm, they will 'master' their pain. Women are not prepared for the pain and they will tell you the next day they never imagined how severe the pain was going to be, but they coped as long as they were able. For many women, the induction of labor and waiting for the magic four centimeters (required by some doctors before an epidural can be placed) is an intolerable length of time to be in excruciating pain."

Ms. Dibal describes the pain of labor to her clients in this way: "It will be the hardest thing you have ever done."

Advice to Moms

"One must prepare as if preparing for a marathon. (A marathon would be easier.) The pain comes in waves, like the tide. It is regular and increases. There comes a time in the labor when all you can remember of the past is pain and the future holds more pain. It is terrifying. That is why you have a support team, to get you through it. There is no weakness in deciding this is not for you and getting the pain medication you need. I think the goal each woman sets for herself needs to be realistic or the feelings of failure can be overwhelming."

Ms. Julia Lange Kessler, a certified midwife at HVO Midwives, Nyack Hospital, New York

"Even the most knowledgeable [meaning educated in childbirth] cannot know how they will respond. But the truth is that you will not get more than you can handle unless you are being given drugs to speed up or augment your labor. It [labor] is not designed to kill you." She described attending another midwife's labor recently, whom she described as "well nourished and very well educated." The midwife described her labor to Ms. Lange Kessler as "grueling." Ms. Lange Kessler concluded, "You can never tell how anyone will respond."

Advice to Moms

"Every woman experiences labor differently. Your attitude, your ability to relax, your pain threshold, nutrition, etc. all make a difference. If you fight the contractions, they are much more painful. If you relax, the contractions are more efficient, and you will experience less of the pain."

This Is What Doulas and Childbirth Educators Told Us

Ms. Penny Simkin, a certified doula, co-founder of DONA International, and author of several books on the topic of pregnancy and childbirth

"Yes and no. My childbirth-class students are prepared to deal with labor pain, and both women and partners are prepared for the sounds and behavior of laboring women. They are not prepared for the exact sensations, however."

"[In preparing first-time moms for the pain of labor] I tell them the pain is severe. It comes and goes. It is not a sign of injury or damage and is manageable without pain medications if the following conditions exist:

1. The woman wants to avoid pain medications.
2. She has excellent support from her caregiving staff, her partner, and a doula.
3. She is educated and prepared in self-help pain relief.
4. She has a reasonably normal labor.

"Most American women today have little confidence that they are able to bear labor pain. They worry that they will lose their composure, yell or scream, writhe, and lose their ability to think or express themselves clearly. They worry about embarrassing themselves, scaring their loved ones, or being judged by the staff. The specter of losing control of their own behavior may be as much of an incentive for women to have an epidural as their fear of pain."

Advice to Moms

"I try to reassure my students and clients that the labor skills I teach will help them maintain their composure while allowing them to behave instinctually. I also try to help the partners understand the woman's behavior without worry. I also suggest that my students and clients know some self-help comforting measures, even if they are planning an epidural, since all hospitals, even those with many anesthesiologists on staff, sometimes have to ask women to wait for an epidural. The wait is sometimes upsetting and frightening for the woman who has no way to help herself."

Ms. Tracy Hartley, a certified doula, and founder and director of B★E★S★T Doula Service, Los Angeles, California

"Many women seem to be surprised by the intensity and level of the pain. No one can really imagine what pain will feel like until they've experienced it. On the other hand, I've had clients say they had been expecting the pain to be much worse than it actually was, while a few have said it was exactly what they thought it would be.

"To describe the pain of labor, I tell my clients that labor pain is different for everyone and that if labor is moving along on a relatively normal progressive track, the pain will most likely not be more than they can handle. I tell them that for some women, it may have the intensity of the pain they feel when they hit their head on an open cabinet door; at first they will think they are going to pass out or throw up, but by the time these thoughts have been processed, the pain is already decreasing and, within a few seconds, the intensity will be tolerable again. I also say that some women have described the pain as being like a leg cramp in their abdomen, but one that doesn't last very long, and that some women feel only menstrual-like cramping."

Advice to Moms

"I provide pregnant women with pain-reduction suggestions such as hypnosis, relaxation, heat, cold, water, and massage, to let them know that they have the tools in their control to help them cope with whatever level of pain they may have."

This Is What Physicians Told Us

Joy Hawkins, M.D., director of obstetric anesthesia, University of Colorado Hospital, Denver, Colorado

Dr. Hawkins points out that women can feel confused by the information available to them. "I find most childbirth education classes tend to downplay pain and assure women they can handle it through breathing, water, focus, etc. This surely contributes to the feelings of failure and dissatisfaction women have when they do need and receive analgesia [pain relief] for labor. Plus it contrasts with the horror stories women hear from family and friends. As a result, many patients are unsure and confused about what to expect."

In her description of labor pain, Dr. Hawkins explains to first-time moms, "Each labor experience is different and unique, so keep an open mind and be flexible."

Advice to Moms

"Educate yourself, know your options, and then decide which options to exercise when the time comes. Everyone around you in labor and delivery is there to help you have a satisfying, safe experience and you can change your mind about your plans any time, including your plans for pain relief."

Ronald Ramus, M.D., an obstetrician at Parkland Memorial Hospital, and associate professor of obstetrics and gynecology, the University of Texas Southwestern Medical Center, Dallas, Texas

"I think there's a tremendous variety of pain perception and assessment in first-time moms. There are definitely cultural and ethnic influences that play a role. The pain of labor is really not something anyone can prepare for. Preconceived notions are huge—if you think it's going to hurt, then it will be excruciating; if you think it can't be that bad, and you are determined to 'handle' the pain on your own, or there are no drugs or anesthesia available, it doesn't seem as bad."

Advice to Moms

Dr. Ramus does not try to explain labor pain to his patients. "I wouldn't know how, but I am extremely sympathetic to any woman who wants help [i.e., drugs] dealing with the pain. In no way is it a sign of anything other than significant pain."

T. Bogard, M.D., an obstetric anesthesiologist, Wake Forest University School of Medicine and Forsyth Medical Center, Winston-Salem, North Carolina

"No, women are not prepared, and few seem curious enough to get literature or go to lectures, perhaps due to fear. Their reluctance to learn more also seems to be promoted by family encouragement (mothers, sisters, grandmothers, etc.) who assure them, 'You'll do fine.' "

Advice to Moms

"I tell [couples] not to discount themselves; they are a lot stronger than they think they are. If husbands and/or mothers are present, I then stress the importance of coaching (without making demands). Finally, I emphasize the importance of our labor nurses as sources of strength, encouragement, and information."

RESOURCES

- americanbaby.com
- www.maternitywise.org (Maternity Center Association)
- Storknet.com
- ePregnancy.com

We suggest the following books and magazines, which provide more information on the topics of fear, pain, and pain management during labor and delivery:

Books
Pregnancy, Childbirth and the Newborn, by Penny Simkin, Janet Whalley, and Ann Keppler (New York: Simon and Schuster, 2001).
Labor Day: Shared Experiences from the Delivery Room, by Ann-Marie Giglio (New York: Workman, 1999).

The Girlfriends' Guide to Pregnancy, Or Everything Your Doctor Won't Tell You, by Vicki Iovine (New York: Pocket Books, 1995).

Magazines
ePregnancy
Pregnancy
FitPregnancy
AmericanBaby

Three

YOUR VERY NORMAL,
VERY COMMON FEARS
OF CHILDBIRTH

Women's fear of childbirth is universal and has been documented in most cultures throughout history. There are several different perspectives on why women experience fear during pregnancy. Some childbirth experts have asserted recently that women *learn* to fear childbirth through cultural messages that often depict dramatic and sensationalized images of birth on television and in the other media. They suggest that this learning process, combined with the prevalence of negative birth stories often told by girlfriends, sisters, and mothers, contributes to and, according to some, even *causes*, women's fear in anticipation of childbirth.

Since women's fears of childbirth existed long before the Discovery Channel's televised birth stories, however, and presumably women have been sharing accounts of their childbirth experience for centuries, it is possible that the fear associated with labor and birth may simply be a natural response to this major life event. In fact, some researchers have suggested that fear during pregnancy is not only common, but *rational*, given that births, even normal births, have always been characterized by "inherent pain and unpredictability."[1]

This perspective suggests that some amount of fear may actually play a positive role during pregnancy by providing motivation for women to prepare for their impending childbirth. In addition to educating yourself on childbirth through books, classes, magazines, and various websites, an important part of this preparation can involve sharing your feelings with other women who are about to give birth, or seeking the support and advice of women who have already "been there, done that."

For most people, *stress* is just a part of everyday modern life, but pregnant women often experience stress that is specifically associated with their pregnancy, on top of all of the other day-to-day stressors. Although pregnancy-related stress is very common, and very normal, it is understandably troubling to women, most of whom are striving to have a positive pregnancy and childbirth experience.

The goal of this section is not to heighten your fears and stress levels by focusing on them, but to assure you that these emotions are common during pregnancy and to provide you with advice on how to manage these feelings. If you are not feeling fearful or stressed at this point in your pregnancy, great! You are off to a positive start. If you find yourself experiencing these emotions, however, or are taking on any of these worries at any point in your pregnancy, it may be helpful to see how common these fears are and read some suggestions that could help you effectively manage your fear and stress levels in anticipation of giving birth.

In this chapter you will learn

- The most common *specific* fears associated with childbirth for first-time and repeat moms.
- How to manage "feeling like a chicken."
- The stress factor—what is normal, and why you and your caregivers should not dismiss excessive fear and stress.
- Ten easy relaxation tips for pregnant women.

A List of the Most Common Fears of First-Time and Repeat Moms

First-Time Moms
First-time moms report more intense fears of childbirth than women who have previously given birth, although many women who have already experienced labor have fears associated with a repeat childbirth.[2] So, for some women, the *less* you know, the more you fear, and for others, the *more* you know, the more you fear. This is not altogether comforting, but it is important for you to know, whether you are expecting your first or your sixth baby, that it is not uncommon to feel a peculiar mix of ecstatic joy, excitement, wonder, and anticipation, combined with feelings of vulnerability, anxiety, and fear.

If this is your *first childbirth,* your fears may typically focus on:

- Worry about labor pain.
- Concern over whether you will actually "be able to do it."
- Fear that there may be something wrong with the baby.
- Worry over loss of dignity.
- Fear of injury to your body during childbirth.
- Concern over the possibility of an emergency cesarean delivery.
- Fear of dying during childbirth.[3]

HOW FIRST-TIME MOMS CAN MANAGE
THESE FEARS

- **If you are worried about labor pain:** Prepare yourself by reading books on childbirth (since you are reading this now, you've already begun to use your coping skills). Investigate the pain-relief options available to you and labor support methods (tubs, massage, birth balls) at your hospital or birth center. Talk about your concerns with your childbirth educator, your caregivers, your partner, and other supportive people in your life. Let others *reassure* you. Learn and *practice* relaxation techniques most suitable to you. They will help with your anxiety and can benefit you during labor.

- **If you are concerned over whether you will actually be able to "do it":** Since most births in the United States occur in a hospital setting, most women have never seen or been a part of another woman's childbirth experience, and as a result many women have a hard time picturing how they will be able to meet this challenge. Childbirth does *not* require previous experience. The fact that you have not given birth before does not mean you will not *know how* to. If you are a first-time mom you may need reassurance that your body is designed to facilitate moving the baby from the comfort of your womb to the outside world.

- **If you are worried that there may be "something wrong" with the baby:** *Most babies* are born without complications. In the United States it is estimated that 4 percent of babies are born with some type of birth defect, and the infant mortality rate (which tracks mortality rates not just for newborns but for babies up to one year of age) is 7 per 1,000 live births.[4] Many women have had a variety of tests during their pregnancy that have already ruled out a number of significant complications. It may allay your concerns to remember that you are giving birth in a setting where you are surrounded by professionals who are ready to handle any unforeseen complication.

- **If you worry about modesty or the possible loss of dignity:** Most people don't relish the idea of being completely exposed to a roomful of strangers, even if it is for the purpose of delivering a baby. Many women are concerned that their privacy or sense of modesty will not be respected, or that during the strain of labor they may be unable to "control" themselves and may behave in a way they would not under ordinary circumstances. It may be hard to believe right now, but as labor gets under way, you may find that you worry a lot less over issues of modesty, and your very desire to stay "in control" may change significantly as you adjust to the physical demands your body makes on you during labor and delivery. Ask your caregivers about this. They will most likely tell you they have seen and heard it all while supporting women during childbirth.

This is not to minimize the importance of having your privacy respected or of needing a sense of control over your own childbirth process, but if you are giving birth in an environment where the labor professionals are attentive to the needs and concerns of birthing mothers, these worries will likely subside once you begin to labor.

- **If you are fearful of injury to your body during childbirth:** Your body is capable of giving birth, and the pain most women will experience during childbirth does *not* mean something is wrong. This, however, does not suggest that you therefore must tolerate the pain, but that you do not need to fear that it is an indicator of anything other than the process of labor.

Some women are specifically worried about the possibility of having an episiotomy (a surgical cut from the vagina to the rectum) during birth. The trend toward giving women routine episiotomies is changing in most hospitals. Physicians are taking a more conservative approach to this procedure, due to an increased recognition that episiotomies can result in a far more painful recovery period for women and in some cases may be associated with more tissue and muscle damage than the vaginal tear it was meant to prevent.

Physicians and midwives can use various methods to avoid an episiotomy. Encouraging women to assume a sitting or side-lying position, or to get into a hands-and-knees position, can help them avoid overdistension (tearing) of the perineum (vaginal and rectal area). Other techniques used to avoid an episiotomy include prenatal massage of the perineal area, controlled and slow delivery of the baby, and perineal support and massage with the use of warm compresses treated with nonfragrant oil as the baby is born.

- **If you have concerns about the possibility of an emergency cesarean delivery:** Find out your hospital's cesarean section rate by asking your obstetrician or the childbirth educator at your hospital. Is it at or below the national average? (The national average is currently approximately 25 percent of all births.) If your physician or hospital handles a large number of women who are considered high risk, their cesarean rate may be higher than those physicians or hospitals who see women who are considered low risk, and therefore less likely to have health conditions that might lead to cesarean deliveries. Ask what your particular physician's cesarean section rate is and factor this in when determining where to give birth and with whom.

- **If you have a fear of dying during childbirth:** Fortunately, the maternal mortality (death rate) in the United States is significantly lower than that of most of the rest of the world. In the last century, the risk of death from complications for pregnant women has decreased by nearly 99 percent, from approximately 850 maternal deaths per 100,000 live births in 1900, to 7 in 100,000 for white women and 18 to 22 in 100,000 for African American women, in the United States today.[5] There are various theories on the reasons for a higher maternal mortality rate among African American women; it is thought that inadequate resources and lack of access to health care services contribute to this disparity.

As a point of comparison, the chances of women dying due to a pregnancy complication in many underdeveloped countries can range from 55 to a staggering 900 maternal deaths per 100,000 live births.[6]

Tokophobia is the extreme anxiety or fear of death during childbirth, which can result in the avoidance of childbirth, even when there is the desire to have children. It is estimated that approximately 6 percent of pregnant women suffer from this condition. It was previously thought that only Western women experienced this psychological condition; however, tokophobia has also been found to exist in other cultures.[7]

At various times during pregnancy women may experience passing feelings of fear or even dread in anticipation of giving birth, but this does *not* mean they are suffering from tokophobia. Women who experience *significant* fear may have "nightmares, physical complaints and feel unable to concentrate on work and family activities."[8]

If you feel that the fear and anxiety you are experiencing are such that you are in need of professional support, your concerns may not be apparent to your obstetrician. According to Diana Dell, M.D., obstetrician and psychiatrist at Duke University, "Obstetrical care providers are quite accustomed to providing reassurance to women who are fearful of childbirth, because milder fears are very common. When fears are more intense, as in tokophobia, women often have to explain this to their caregiver and ask for psychological consultation when needed."

Regarding women's fears in anticipation of childbirth, Dr. Dell offers some reassuring words: "If women don't have at least *some* fears or concerns about childbirth, they are probably not adequately prepared. Until fairly recently in our history, childbirth was fraught with many hazards; it is likely that fears associated with childbirth are somehow hardwired into our DNA."

Repeat Moms

If you are a repeat mom, your fears may typically focus on:

- Worry about labor pain.
- Worry about moments of loss of control during labor and birth.
- Fear of dying during childbirth.[9]

Fear of a repeat childbirth experience can take months or even years to surface, and the fear may not appear until a subsequent pregnancy. Women who have previously experienced a labor that resulted in an emergency cesarean delivery, a long and difficult labor, or the use of forceps to extract the baby have shown high levels of fear and anxiety associated with another childbirth.[10]

Labor pain itself can contribute to women developing fear of another delivery. Some women who had no significant fear of childbirth during their first pregnancy, but who encountered a difficult first labor and delivery, have developed severe fear of giving birth again.[11]

HOW REPEAT MOMS CAN MANAGE THESE FEARS:

- **If you are worried about labor pain:** If your previous birth experience was difficult or painful, you may worry that you will go through a similar ordeal with this birth. This is certainly a reasonable apprehension, given what you've been through, but it may help you to keep in mind that *every* labor and delivery experience is different. Women who have had a difficult and painful birth with one baby can go on to have a relatively easy birth with another, and the reverse can be true as well. If pain control was an issue in the past, make your caregivers aware of this and ask if there is something that can be done differently this time around. Since no two births are alike, there is a good chance this labor and delivery will *not* be exactly like your previous childbirth experience(s).

- **If you are worried about loss of control:** Control during childbirth can mean different things to different people. To some women, even repeat moms, the concern may be about losing control of yourself physically, in response to the demands of labor. Concern over control can also reflect apprehension regarding other issues during childbirth: control over timing of pain-relief choices, control over who can join you in the delivery room, control over whether you can eat or drink during labor, and a variety of other issues that may concern you.

  If your previous childbirth was marked by control issues that left you feeling dissatisfied, talk with your caregivers about your specific concerns. If you did not have someone other than your partner in the delivery room with you before, and you think you might benefit from more support this time around, you may want to consider asking a friend or hiring a doula or midwife to help you during labor.

- **If you have a fear of dying during childbirth:** Whether you are a first-time or repeat mom, our advice is the same (see page 58), but you now have the advantage of having already experienced childbirth to help you keep things in perspective. Presumably you came out of the experience like most women do: strong and healthy enough to do it again!

How to Manage Feeling Like a Chicken

Speak Up
You may feel uncomfortable at the thought of talking openly about your fears of childbirth with your caregivers. Sometimes women experience a sense of shame about their own negative feelings toward childbirth and are reluctant to reveal these feelings to others for various reasons. Your doctor or caregiver may appear too busy to have the time to address your fear and anxi-

ety, or you may worry about being perceived as a "difficult" patient by exposing your vulnerable feelings. If your physician or caregiver has not specifically addressed how you may be feeling regarding the pain involved in labor and delivery, whether you are a first-time mom or a repeat mom, you may have to raise this issue yourself.

We encourage you not to conceal your fears from your doctor and caregivers; instead, talk honestly and openly about these emotions. Even if you are unable to pinpoint exactly what you fear about the experience of labor and delivery (the fear of pain itself is enough), just talking with your physician or caregiver about your generalized feelings of concern, anxiety, or fearfulness will help ease your mind. Your doctor and caregivers need to understand your fears and concerns before they can attempt to help you develop successful coping strategies.

You may also find it reassuring to arrange a meeting with an anesthesiologist to discuss your concerns regarding pain during labor. He or she will be able to inform you of the medical options that are available for pain relief during the various stages of labor, and can describe how you will be involved in the decision-making process.

If your preference is to avoid the use of drugs, you may take comfort in contacting other women who have had a medication-free birth. Ask them about the pain-management techniques they used and how they managed to cope with their own labor pain. Find out more about the birth philosophies that offer support and resources to women who wish to have a medication-free birth (see chapter six).

As you will see in our birth stories (chapter ten) and in our caregiver interviews (chapter eleven), it is to your benefit to learn about your medical pain-relief options even if you are undecided about whether you will use medications, and even if you are adamant that you won't. If at some point during labor you decide you need medications, or if there is an unlikely emergency situation, you will feel better prepared if you are informed about the medications being used and how they will affect both you and your newborn.

Listen—If It's True, It's Not a Horror Story

Listen to other women whom you trust to give you a realistic account of the pain they experienced during labor, what they found effective for pain relief, and how they dealt with their fears and anxieties before and during childbirth. We often hear of difficult birth experiences referred to as horror stories, and some people feel it is impolite or inappropriate to reveal graphic details of the pain they endured during childbirth. But to dismiss a woman's account of her difficult labor and delivery as a horror story does not honor her birth experience. Often these stories are simply truthful accounts of women's painful and difficult births.

One woman's description of her especially difficult birth may, in fact, be your opportunity to prepare yourself by gathering information from your caregivers about all of the safe options for pain relief available to you in your hospital or birth center prior to your own childbirth experience. It may also provide you with the knowledge you need in order to have a dialogue with your physician or caregiver regarding various complications that may arise and how they would handle them in a worst-case-scenario situation. Keep in mind that some women's reports of disappointing birth experiences are based on the difficulty they had with caregivers who did not offer appropriate "alternative" pain-management interventions and were resistant to the laboring woman's preference to *avoid* epidural and narcotic interventions.

Hearing from other women about their impressions, fears, emotions, sensations, and intense pain provides you with information and a perspective that will allow you to work with your physician and caregivers to prepare for your own unique and satisfying childbirth experience.

Don't forget that you will also hear from many women who had nontraumatic, satisfying, and wonderful birth experiences, some of whom benefited from the relief of narcotics and epidurals and some who opted for absolutely no pharmacological pain relief. Even if you feel you'll want every type of pain relief the anesthesiologist has to offer once labor begins, stories from women who had beautiful and satisfying *natural* births may provide you with inspiration and encouragement during your own labor.

Visit the Hospital or Birth Center

Many hospitals and birth centers encourage women to tour the maternity unit or birthing suites prior to their due date. It is advantageous to *see* and *hear* what a maternity unit is all about before you get there. During your tour you may see things that reassure you, or you may even experience sights and sounds that are foreign and possibly intimidating. This is why you are there! It is vital that you get a realistic view of what happens in your chosen facility, to help you understand what it will be like when it is your time to give birth.

If the tour itself raises any questions or contributes to your sense of anxiety, raise these specific concerns and work through them with your caregiver. The goal of this tour is for you to develop a sense of familiarity with your future birth environment. If you are able to form an impression of the sights, sounds, and sensations of the birthing unit, your anxiety level may be reduced when you arrive for the real thing.

Seek Professional Help

If your physician or caregiver does not seem sympathetic or responsive to your concerns, or if you feel your fear and anxiety exceed what you normally experience during stressful life events, consider meeting with a different obstetric caregiver. A doula, midwife, obstetrician, social worker, or psychologist can listen, provide encouragement, and help you develop effective coping strategies to use during labor and delivery.

Are Women Making Plans to Avoid Labor Pain?

Fear of labor pain may contribute to the recent increase in the number of elective, or prescheduled, cesarean deliveries.[12] The debate about this controversial issue continues, with many physicians and childbirth advocates urging women and their obstetricians not to opt for an elective cesarean delivery without clinical justification; a cesarean delivery, while sometimes a lifesaving procedure for both mother and newborn carries with it risks inherent to most major surgical interventions.

Not all women who opt for elective cesarean delivery do so out of anxiety associated with labor pain, of course. Some choose cesarean delivery because of concern of possible complications that may result from vaginal delivery, such as pelvic-floor injury or sexual dysfunction, worry over potential harm to the baby during labor and delivery (due to a specific aspect of the pregnancy or fetal development, such as an especially large baby), and a desire for an electively timed delivery to work around the mother's or doctor's schedule.

Choosing a cesarean delivery as a way to eliminate labor pain altogether may emphasize the need for better communication between pregnant women and their caregivers around issues of fear and anxiety in anticipation of childbirth. It may also suggest the need for increased resources devoted to identifying women who have significant fear and anxiety during pregnancy, and it may raise important concerns regarding the effectiveness of pain management during labor.

THE STRESS FACTOR DURING PREGNANCY

There is stress; then there is high stress. Stress is a part of most major life events, even *positive* life events like a pregnancy. Fortunately, most women are able to adjust to the new stressors associated with their pregnancy. Some women, however, may not cope well with this additional stress.

TYPICAL STRESSORS FOR PREGNANT WOMEN

Studies suggest that pregnant women are most concerned about the following issues during pregnancy:

"Medical problems, physical symptoms, parenting/relationships, bodily changes, labor and delivery, and the health of the baby."[13]

Anxiety exists throughout pregnancy in general, but typically increases and is most significant in your last trimester.[14] Feelings of *significant* anxiety during pregnancy and childbirth may do more than just produce emotional discomfort for women; severe stress during pregnancy has actually been associated with pregnancy complications. Studies suggest a link between high levels of maternal stress and complications with fetal development.[15]

FACTORS THAT CAN CAUSE HIGH STRESS DURING PREGNANCY

Excessive stress during pregnancy not only potentially impacts the newborn, but can impact the pregnant woman as well. Women under significant amounts of stress may experience symptoms including fatigue, sleeplessness, anxiety, poor appetite or overeating, headaches, and backaches. Below we list several factors that are believed to cause or contribute to more extreme forms of stress during pregnancy.

Previous Miscarriage and Late-Pregnancy Loss

Women who have miscarried or experienced the loss of an infant report increased levels of fear and anxiety during subsequent pregnancies. In particular, women who had a late-pregnancy miscarriage or loss of an infant have been shown to experience more anxiety in their next pregnancy than women who have never experienced such a loss.[16]

Those dealing with heightened anxiety during pregnancy as a result of such a loss need to communicate this to their caregivers. Women dealing with this loss should expect their caregivers to be sensitive to their unique concerns and provide reassurance throughout their pregnancy, including recommending additional support to them and to their partners, if necessary.

High-Risk Pregnancy and Bed Rest

Women dealing with a high-risk pregnancy and confined to bed rest, whether at home or in a hospital, face an exceptional number of stressors, often all at once. Women who are hospitalized during this time must deal with the emotional strain of being separated from their home and partners (or other children), combined with the stress of living in the institutionalized setting of a hospital. Women on bed rest often report feelings of helplessness, loss of control, endless boredom, loneliness, and ongoing worry for the health of their unborn baby. Those who are given medications for preterm labor may also be worried about the effects of these drugs on their infants.[17]

Professionals who work with women confined to bed rest emphasize the need for strong social support and effective coping mechanisms to help them get through this extraordinarily difficult and stressful (but temporary) time in their lives. Some of the suggestions caregivers often provide to women on bed rest include encouraging visits from family and friends and planning activities to relieve boredom throughout the day. Now's the time to catch up on your favorite sitcoms or talk shows, something your non–bed rest pregnant friends can envy. For women confined to a hospital bed during this time, caregivers recommend that you wear your own clothing rather than hospital gowns to reduce the feeling of being in the role of "sick patient." Experts and moms previously confined to bed rest recommend that women take a one-day-at-a-time countdown approach and remind themselves that in spite of *feeling* unproductive by remaining on bed rest, they are actually *being* productive, by doing what's best for the baby.

Fortunately, there is now an active Internet community of moms on bed rest who support one another "virtually" via their computer. Various chat rooms, support groups, and websites containing educational information specifically for pregnant women on bed rest have been created over the last few years and many women have found these resources vital to keeping them sane during this time (see resources at the end of this chapter).

Domestic or Emotional Abuse

Women who are victims of domestic or sexual abuse suffer from increased levels of stress that can impact their overall emotional state during pregnancy.[18] Women's memories of previous victimization can also cause increased fear and anxiety during pregnancy and childbirth.[19]

Many physicians, in their initial health assessment of pregnant women, now routinely ask their patients whether there are any domestic abuse issues or concerns. These very personal issues are often difficult for women to discuss with others, but if you are a victim of abuse, or have a history of abuse, your caregivers need to be aware of these concerns in order to provide the reassurance and appropriate resources you may need.

Given the suggested connection between high stress during pregnancy and potential negative clinical outcomes, it is vital that you and your caregivers pay attention to how you are feeling during your pregnancy in anticipation of your impending childbirth experience.

Why You (and Your Caregivers) Should Not
Dismiss Excessive Fear and Stress

> **DID YOU KNOW?** *In some women whose stress levels rise significantly, the health risks to themselves and their newborns may also increase.*[20] Very high *levels of stress in pregnant women may increase the risk of preterm labor and low-birth-weight babies. Even babies born full term to women who suffer from high levels of stress and anxiety are more likely to be born with a low birth weight.*[21]

TIPS FOR HOW TO MANAGE YOUR STRESS LEVEL DURING PREGNANCY

Start Slimming Down . . . Your Calendar

By decreasing or eliminating some of the stressors over which you have control, your overall stress level may also decrease. For example, if you are stressed by staying involved in activities at your prepregnancy pace, you may benefit by reducing your activity level to better match your energy level. Identify the stressors that you find most taxing and, if possible, find ways to reduce or get rid of them, at least for the next few months. This may help you keep your overall stress level in check.

Focus on What You Are Able to Control

Another approach to keeping your stress level to a minimum is to simply not *focus* on all of the possible unknowns and what-ifs and instead *stay focused* on the aspects of your pregnancy over which you do have control, such as getting enough rest, exercise, and good nutrition, in addition to learning about the many childbirth preparation techniques and pain-relief options available to you on your baby's birth day.

If You Can't Control the Situation, Control Your Response to the Situation

Often, it is not the source of stress but how you manage the stressful situation that determines the difference between feeling as if you are coping and feeling anxious and overwhelmed. Sometimes it is not possible to eliminate the source of stress. In this case, another effective stress buster involves attempting to alter the intensity of your *response* to the stressors.

When you find yourself feeling nervous or stressed, try to pinpoint the exact thoughts you were having that stirred up those feelings in the first place. Then actively stop the thoughts that caused those negative feelings. Replace them with thoughts about some other topic that will promote calmer or more neutral feelings. Some people have compared this to changing the tape in your VCR: Your thoughts are the tapes. If you don't like how they make you feel, press STOP, insert another one, and press START.

This requires some practice and you may learn this technique, and others, in your childbirth preparation classes. By being conscious of the stressful thoughts you are having, then *replacing* these thoughts with more positive ones, you may notice a decrease in your stress level.

A Quick and Simple Relaxation Plan for Moms-to-Be

Strategies that reduce your stress not only help you rest better and feel better throughout your pregnancy, but may also help to prepare you emotionally and physically for a positive childbirth experience. And, if nothing else, women who make an effort to use healthy coping skills may be less likely to slip into unhealthy ways of dealing with the increased stress of pregnancy, such as overeating, smoking, and drinking alcohol.

Research has suggested that relaxation techniques used throughout pregnancy not only benefit women during labor and delivery, but may also enhance fetal development. James McCubbin, Ph.D., professor and chair of psychology at Clemson University in Clemson, South Carolina, has devised an easy ten-point relaxation plan for pregnant women:

1. Relax and do the things you enjoy for your health and the baby's: read, knit, walk, or listen to music.
2. If taking time to relax each day does not come naturally to you, schedule "baby time" in your planner and consistently keep that slot free just for yourself.
3. Get comfortable. A quiet room with no phone works best. Lying down or reclining is good. Lie slightly tilted to one side with your belly (and baby) partially supported by a pillow.
4. Prepare mentally. Clear your mind of distractions and focus on your relaxation.
5. Control the relaxation you give to your body and your baby. Chores can wait; deadlines may need to be loosened. Your relaxation is not a luxury; it is a necessity.
6. Focus on your breathing. Use slow, steady, deep breaths from your belly, not your chest.
7. Locate the tension. Where specifically is your body feeling stress? Your neck? Lower back? Learn to identify where you are feeling tension and then . . .
8. Release the tension in each muscle group. Pay attention to the sensation of the tension dissolving when you relax muscles in different parts of your body.
9. Imagine yourself in your favorite restful place—maybe on the beach, by a stream, or on a mountaintop. Challenge your senses to "hear," "smell," and "see" where you have chosen to relax.
10. Practice and enjoy the pleasant feelings you have given yourself and your baby and try to practice these steps daily for at least twenty to thirty minutes. Relax *throughout* your pregnancy, for yourself and for your baby.

RESOURCES

For general information on pregnancy and birth, including issues related to emotional health during pregnancy: www.modimes.org. (March of Dimes).

For excellent information specifically for moms on bed rest, or moms with a high-risk pregnancy: www.sidelines.org.

Or read:

The Pregnancy Bed Rest Book: A Survival Guide for Expectant Mothers and Their Families, by Amy E. Tracy (New York: Berkley Books, 2001).

For more information on the effects of sexual abuse on childbirth, read:

When Survivors Give Birth: Understanding and Healing the Effects of Early Sexual Abuse on Childbearing Women, by Penny Simkin and Phyllis Klaus (Seattle, Washington: Classic Day Publishing, 2004).

Four

FULL-THROTTLE
PAIN RELIEF

Techniques That Can *Eliminate*
Your Labor Pain

Most women would prefer to experience as little pain as possible during childbirth. Some might admit they would prefer to experience no pain at all. Although an entirely pain-free birth is not yet possible, you *are* now able to experience childbirth with less pain than ever before. One way to achieve this is by using the best pain-relief medicine available today.

> **DID YOU KNOW?** *In the United States over half of the 4 million women a year who give birth (2.4 million) use an epidural for pain relief during labor.*

Contrary to information you may have read or heard, it is *not* accurate to suggest you must choose between *comfort* and *safety* when determining the type of pain management you prefer during childbirth. There are risks involved in the everyday use of *all* safe and effective forms of modern technology or modern medicine; for example, whether it's our daily use of modern transportation, or taking the birth control pill to prevent pregnancy, there is a certain amount of risk tolerated in exchange for the benefits of modern life. Similarly, there is some risk involved in the use of modern medicine for the purpose of pain relief during childbirth.

Most moms (and anesthesiologists) will tell you that the *worst* time to try to grasp all of your options and weigh the risks and benefits of pain-relief medications is in the middle of a contraction. You don't need to choose which specific medications or techniques you want to use *before* you go into labor, but you should have a general understanding about the advantages and disadvantages of the most commonly used medications before you are faced with making pain-relief decisions in the labor and delivery room.

The definitions provided below will help you understand the difference between the medical pain-relief methods that are described in the next few chapters.

The epidural is known as "regional anesthesia" since its pain relief affects only the specific region of the body where the medication is administered. The epidural involves the insertion of a needle that threads a small, thin catheter into your lower spine; the epidural catheter remains in place until after you give birth. Pain-relief medications are administered via the epidural throughout your labor. Variations on the epidural are becoming increasingly popular on maternity units, including the *combined spinal epidural* (CSE) and the *patient-controlled epidural analgesia* (PCEA). These are described in detail in this chapter. The CSE and PCEA are the most effective medical pain-relief methods used during childbirth in most hospitals.

The spinal (or spinal block) is also known as "regional anesthesia." It is also administered with a needle into your lower spine, but its effects are more immediate than an epidural's, and no catheter is inserted for continued pain relief. The spinal is almost exclusively used for a cesarean delivery or at the end of labor if it appears that forceps—

a device used to assist the baby out of the birth canal—
may be needed to deliver the baby.

General anesthesia is rarely used during childbirth, usually
only in cases involving an emergency situation with the
mother or baby. General anesthetics (medicines that
completely eliminate sensation by producing a state of
sleep during labor or birth) can be administered quickly,
and the effects are almost instantaneous.

In this section we describe:

- Exactly what an epidural is, how the procedure is
  done, and how it eliminates your labor pain.
- The newer forms of epidurals that are gaining
  popularity with women and caregivers: *combined spinal
  epidural (CSE)* and *patient-controlled epidural analgesia
  (PCEA)*.
- The risks and side effects of all forms of the epidural.
- The concerns and controversy surrounding the use of
  the epidural during childbirth.
- Perspectives of women and caregivers on the
  experience of using an epidural during childbirth.

THE EPIDURAL

What It Is and What It Does

An epidural is an injection of pain-relief medications into your
lower spine. The epidural, also called epidural analgesia (analgesia means pain reducer), as a pain-relief option for women during childbirth has been around since the 1950s, but an epidural
given to women during childbirth today is very different than
an epidural given even ten years ago. Refinements in the last
decade have resulted in a better overall experience for women,
giving them better control and, in some cases, more mobility
than past epidurals allowed. The epidural has improved in both

safety and effectiveness in the last decade and is now one of the most popular pain-relief methods for women giving birth in hospitals. The medications in the epidural reduce or completely eliminate your labor pain by blocking your sensations from the waist down. Within ten to twenty minutes or less, epidural analgesia, when successfully administered, can eliminate most or all of your labor pain.

TAKE A MESSAGE PLEASE . . .

The epidural relieves pain by blocking the nerves that carry pain sensations from the uterus and cervix to your brain. The medications given in the epidural prevent these pain messages from traveling through your spinal cord to your brain.

How It Is Done and How It Feels

An epidural involves placing a needle into the epidural space (the space between the spinal bone and the spinal cord) that surrounds the lower part of your spinal cord. Since the needle is placed *below* the spinal cord, there is almost no risk of mistakenly hitting the cord itself during placement. After taking your medical history, the anesthesiologist will briefly explain to you how the procedure will be done. You will be asked to curl up into a ball-like position while lying on your side or sitting at the edge of the bed, and the anesthesiologist will prepare you for placement of the epidural. The procedure typically takes about ten to fifteen minutes from start to finish and you will need to remain still.

Ouch? Ahhh!

Although it sounds painful, most women discover that getting an epidural is less painful than they anticipated, and they prefer the short-term discomfort of the procedure for the almost immediate and long-lasting pain relief.

Often women worry that they won't be able to sit still long enough to get an epidural. Rest assured, doctors, nurses, and midwives expect and understand that this may be a challenge and will help you through the process. Using a position known as the pelvic tilt, commonly taught in childbirth preparation courses, can be a very helpful technique. In this position you lower your head forward, curling your body to form the letter *C* with your back. Tightening your buttock muscles or gently hissing with an open mouth to tighten your abdominal muscles can help you assume this position. The pelvic tilt can also be done either sitting or lying in bed. (By the way, these are excellent exercises anyway to tone and firm your back and abdominal muscles.)

Before you are given an epidural, your anesthesiologist will need to know the following things about you:

- Have you had any food or drink in the last several hours? (If you have just had a meal, this does not disqualify you from getting the epidural, but no solid food once the epidural is in place.)
- Do you have a history of difficulty breathing or any other problems after anesthesia?
- Do you have a history of lower-back problems?
- Is there a family history of problems after anesthesia or surgery?
- Do you have any respiratory problems such as asthma, bronchitis, or pneumonia?

- Do you currently have a cold, sore throat, or the flu?
- Have there been any complications with this pregnancy or with previous pregnancies?
- Do you take any medications, including herbal supplements or over-the-counter medications?

YOUR EPIDURAL STEP BY STEP: HOW IT IS DONE AND HOW IT FEELS

Step one: You will be given an IV to provide your body with extra fluids that can help prevent a fall in blood pressure. You may also be given an antacid and an antinausea medication through the IV to decrease your stomach acid and prevent you from vomiting and experiencing nausea.

Step two: Your back will be wiped with a cool antiseptic solution and a sterile drape will be placed over your lower back.

Step three: A numbing medication will be injected quickly with a tiny needle into the skin on your back where the epidural needle will be inserted. This may feel like a small pinch, no more intense than what you may feel when receiving numbing medication during a dental visit. You may be given a minute or two to wait for the numbing to take effect.

Step four: The epidural needle is inserted into your lower back and it guides a small, narrow plastic tube called a catheter into your spine (epidural space). Since your lower back is now numb, the insertion of the epidural needle feels like pressure on your spine. You may feel a little *zing* or funny-bone sensation when the epidural catheter is inserted. This lasts only a few seconds and is common. A small test amount of medication will be injected to make sure you do not have an adverse reaction to the medication. The anesthesiologist may ask you if you are experiencing any of the following sensations: dizziness, a funny taste in your mouth, numbness of your tongue, or rapid heartbeat. Some women report briefly feeling a cold sensation in their lower back when the medicine first enters their body.

Step five: The needle is removed and the catheter remains in place. The catheter is the tube through which the pain-relief medication can now be given. At this point all you will feel is the tape on your back that holds the catheter in place. Since only a small amount of medication is given to you at any one time, the tube is connected to an automatic pump that delivers your medications on a time-release basis, every hour or so. The amount of medications you receive can be adjusted depending on your needs.

Step six: Your anesthesiologist may ask you to rate your pain level on a scale of one to ten. This provides the anesthesiologist with an indication of how effectively the drugs are working and whether they are adequately relieving your pain. Once it is determined by you and the anesthesiologist that the epidural is doing its thing, and you are now comfortable, the procedure is complete.

You and your baby will be monitored from this point on, until your baby's birth. Your own heart rate and blood pressure will be monitored and your nurse, midwife, or doctor will monitor your baby's heart rate through an electronic fetal monitor. The frequency and intensity of your contractions will also be recorded throughout labor by a device called a tocodynamometer. This device lets your caregivers know how your labor is progressing. Both the electronic fetal monitor (for the baby) and the tocodynamometer (for you) are beltlike bands worn around your belly.

The epidural can be used for as long as you need it. If you feel your pain is returning, let your nurse and doctor know (they will be checking with you throughout your labor to assess your comfort and progress) and your medication can be adjusted. Typically, once the epidural is placed, the catheter is not removed until shortly after you give birth, allowing for medications to be given for the remainder of the labor, birth, and for a short time after the birth of the baby, if necessary. The removal of the epidural catheter is entirely painless. Your doctor simply lifts the tape that holds the tube on your back and gently removes the catheter.

Within a few hours the medications wear off and you fully regain normal sensations in your lower body. At this point it is likely you will be sore and may experience some pain. If you are still in need of pain relief let your nurse or physician know, and you may be given oral pain-relief medication.

Medications Used in an Epidural

The medications used in an epidural can vary, but typically an epidural consists of a small amount of a local anesthetic, usually bupivacaine or ropivacaine, and a small amount of a narcotic, typically fentanyl. You may also receive a dose of Duramorph, which is morphine. This medication will give you complete pain relief that lasts even after the epidural is removed, throughout the hours immediately following the birth of your baby.

Blood levels of morphine found in women who have received Duramorph are extraordinarily low. The possible side effects of this medication are similar to the side effects of narcotics administered by other methods and can include nausea, vomiting, and itching. These side effects are usually minimal, however, since the medication is given in a low dose. A *very rare* side effect of Duramorph is slowing of your breathing, which can occur many hours after the dose is given. For this reason, your nurses will be checking you at regular intervals, for about twenty-four hours after you give birth.

When Can You Get an Epidural?
"Timing is everything," as they say. Just ask a woman in labor who wants relief *now.*

> **DID YOU KNOW?** *Recent research has shown that women who receive an epidural early in labor* do not *have an increased risk of cesarean or instrumental delivery.*[1]

Opinions differ among physicians concerning *when* you should receive an epidural. This is an issue of some importance if your early labor starts off with a bang. If your labor is intense and your pain-coping methods are not keeping the pain manageable, you may want to receive an epidural sooner rather than later. Hospitals and individual physicians may have their own policies or practices regarding the timing of epidurals, and you should be aware of and understand those guidelines or rules before you get to the hospital. Many hospitals and physicians are relatively flexible on this matter and will work with you to determine when it is best to receive various kinds of medications.

A variety of factors may impact the timing of your epidural, including the position of the baby in the birth canal, whether this is your first baby or a repeat birth, and the presence of certain medical issues, such as respiratory or cardiac conditions. Some physicians require the laboring mother to reach four or five centimeters of cervical dilation before they will begin an epidural, out of concern for increasing the chances of a forceps or cesarean delivery. Research does not support this concern, however, and many caregivers feel that whenever women feel they are ready for pain relief, even in early labor, they should be provided with the option of an epidural rather than waiting until they have dilated to a specific number of centimeters.

Does Your Physician Need to Dial Down the Epidural Medication So You Can Push? Not So Fast!

Some physicians cut back on or stop the flow of epidural medications when women reach the pushing stage of labor to avoid increasing the chances of needing to use forceps or vacuum extraction to deliver the baby. However, it has not been demonstrated that this practice actually prevents an increased use of forceps or vacuum extraction. But, not surprisingly, it *does* dramatically increase pain.

Some anesthesiologists taper down the medications as you progress toward the pushing stage of labor, with the idea that you will push more effectively if your sensations are not numbed. Others feel this causes too much pain and is unnecessary as long as your contractions are strong and you are able to push with assistance.

One recent analysis of several studies on this topic concluded:

"There is insufficient evidence to support the hypothesis that discontinuing epidural analgesia late in labor reduces the rate of instrumental delivery, and women should be informed of the risks and benefits of discontinuing epidural analgesia, *and encouraged to participate in the decision of whether to discontinue or not.*"[2]

For some women, the numbness caused by the epidural can make the pushing stage of labor more of a challenge, whereas for other women the pain relief provided by the epidural lets them push more freely, without reservation, rather than trying to push against the pain.

There are ways your caregivers can work with you to assist your pushing efforts if your epidural has dulled your urge to push. Techniques created specifically to assist women in this stage of labor have been developed by obstetric caregivers as epidural usage has increased. These tricks of the trade may include earlier usage of oxytocin to increase the effectiveness of your contractions and prevent dystocia (failure to progress), or increasing the acceptable time limits for the pushing stage of labor. This allows you to rest while fully dilated, until your urge to push returns or until the baby has descended farther into the birth canal. Your caregivers may also assist by helping you reposition (using upright postures or squatting) and cueing you to bear down with the timing of each contraction. You may want to discuss this timing issue with your obstetrician or your anesthesiologist before your due date.

Is It Ever Too Late to Get an Epidural?

Another timing issue often comes up for women who request an epidural toward the end of their labor. Some physicians are reluctant to provide women with an epidural if they are dilated eight or more centimeters. The thinking behind this is that toward the end of labor, due to the intensity of your contractions, it may be difficult for you to sit still for placement of the epidural or that the birth may take place before the numbing medication has a chance to work. With effort and support of your caregivers, it is possible, although often challenging, to remain in position long enough to receive an epidural for the short remainder of your labor; although there *is* the possibility that the baby will arrive before the medication takes effect, there is also the chance that your labor will last longer than predicted and a late epidural may indeed make all the difference as you head into the home stretch.

Some women at this point in their labor are told that to receive an epidural so close to the birth of their baby will not be worth it, since there may only be another fifteen or twenty minutes of pain to deal with. Many women (and caregivers) find this rationalization unacceptable, and some point out that no other patient experiencing intense pain in a hospital setting would be told to endure extreme pain for another fifteen to twenty minutes.

Receiving an epidural at the end of a particularly long and

painful labor can help an exhausted mom rest a bit so she can push more effectively when the time is right for pushing. It can often give women the second wind needed to avoid a cesarean and complete their vaginal birth.

Fortunately, many anesthesiologists are willing to give a woman an epidural upon her request right up to the end, until she has reached the point where the baby's head is crowning (visible).

Reasons You May Choose to Have an Epidural

- You have a strong preference to give birth with as little pain as possible.
- Your other pain-relief medications are not adequately keeping up with the intensity of your labor.
- Nonmedical pain-relief techniques have not sufficiently reduced your pain.
- You're giving birth to a large baby.
- You are having twins, which may increase your chances of needing a cesarean if there is a complication with the birth of one (or both) of the babies. Having an epidural already in place will be to your advantage if an emergency cesarean is needed.
- You've just been given Pitocin to speed up or intensify your labor.
- You've had a long, difficult labor but want to continue to labor some more to try to avoid a cesarean section.
- You are "stuck" (not dilating) and need complete relaxation.
- You need to rest or sleep and cannot do either without adequate pain relief.
- You want *continuous* pain relief instead of having injections every few hours to try to keep ahead of the pain.

*Conditions That May Prevent You from
Having an Epidural*

- You have a history of blood clotting or take certain medications that can affect blood clotting. You should discuss all of this with your obstetrician or an anesthesiologist prior to going into labor.
- You have certain neurological disorders.
- You have previously had certain lower-back surgical procedures.
- During childbirth you prefer to avoid the use of anything more high-tech than the massage setting on your showerhead.

What *You May Feel (or Not) When the Epidural Kicks In*

Many women report partial or no sensation from their tummy down to their toes once the epidural takes effect. Some women describe feeling tightening sensations with each contraction but no pain or discomfort. The amount of sensation you feel after receiving an epidural depends upon how much medication is used in the epidural. Your legs may feel numb and heavy at first; this is common and will subside shortly after you give birth.

How *You May Feel When the Epidural Kicks In*

Relief! Rest! Relaxation! These are a few of the feelings you may experience. The epidural numbs your contractions, *not* your emotions. Once the epidural is in place, most women still feel very much connected with their childbirth experience while feeling disconnected from their labor pain.

Studies have shown that mothers who had an epidural are more comfortable during labor and birth and are more satisfied with their pain-relief choice than women who opted for IV or oral pain relievers during childbirth.[3]

You may find, however, that just because your pain is gone, it does not mean you are stress-free. Some women feel exhausted, especially if they have had a particularly difficult or long labor up to the point of the epidural. Some may still feel worried that their pain will return or anxious about the next phase of labor—birth. Even when these factors are present, many women find that the epidural provides the relief they need to catch up on rest and conserve energy, both emotional and physical, for the next stage of labor.

What Your Partner Can Do

Your partner may stay with you while the epidural is being placed, or he may be asked to wait outside for a few minutes while the procedure takes place. If you feel more comfortable with your partner's support while getting the epidural, let your anesthesiologist or labor nurse know. If he does stay with you when you receive the epidural, he can help by physically assisting you into position for the procedure and by providing emotional comfort and support while the epidural is being administered.

If your partner has joined you in your childbirth preparation courses and is very well informed about how a laboring woman responds to the demands of childbirth (which makes him very unique indeed), he may be less likely to experience heightened anxiety as your labor progresses.

Once the epidural is doing its job and you are resting comfortably, your partner may consider slipping out to the hospital cafeteria after working up a hearty appetite watching you do all the hard work, or he may wisely decide to stay close by and provide emotional support and care while you prepare to enter the next phase of labor. Just because your pain has left you does not mean your labor support should also disappear. You still need encouragement, comfort, and companionship while preparing for the next step and best part of this whole process—the arrival of your baby.

Potential Benefits of the Epidural
During Childbirth

- You will experience complete and rapid pain relief.
- You will remain fully alert; the medications will not make you feel drowsy.
- The epidural is useful for treating especially painful and prolonged labors and relieves painful back labor effectively.
- The elimination of pain allows you to rest and conserve energy.
- The medications in an epidural can be decreased if you are managing well, or increased for better relief if contractions become more severe.
- If a cesarean delivery is determined necessary, or a complication arises, the epidural is already in place and is safer than using general anesthesia.
- If you have a vaginal tear or have an episiotomy, more pain-relief medications can be added to the epidural to provide continued pain relief for several hours *after* you give birth.
- You may benefit from an epidural during childbirth if you have certain heart or lung conditions.
- Women with preeclampsia (high blood pressure) can benefit by the use of an epidural during childbirth: the epidural can help control blood pressure and may help to avoid the use of general anesthesia, which is especially dangerous for women with preeclampsia.

Potential Limitations of Using an
Epidural for Pain Relief

Most women who choose to use an epidural during childbirth are satisfied with the pain relief it brings. Although the success rate is very high, epidurals are sometimes not 100 percent effective, and there are procedures that may accompany the use of the epidural.

- Inadequate anesthesia occurs in approximately 10 to 15 percent of women who receive an epidural.[4]

Breakthrough pain results when the epidural does not fully take effect, sometimes resulting in inadequate pain relief or partial pain relief (when pain relief takes effect on only one side of your body). This can often be corrected by adjusting the medication or by reinserting the epidural needle.

- You will need to have an IV inserted to give your body fluids, which will help keep your blood pressure stable.
- You may need to have a urinary catheter placed in your urethra to catch urine if you are unable to urinate on your own (this can be done *after* the epidural is placed, so you will not feel it, and it is typically removed just before birth).
- Many modern epidurals use smaller doses of medications and will not *completely* block your ability to remain mobile, but due to limited sensation in your legs, you may need to stay in your birthing room or in bed throughout the rest of labor and birth.
- You will need to have continuous monitoring of yourself (with a tocodynamometer) and the baby (with an electronic fetal monitor).

THE ODDS ARE ON YOUR SIDE

Only 1 percent of women who receive an epidural have a complication that leads to severe headache. In the rare cases when the epidural needle goes beyond the epidural space, it can result in an extremely painful headache, but the condition can be successfully treated by taking a small amount of blood from your arm and injecting it into the epidural site to "patch up" the tiny hole created by the epidural needle. This is a common worry but an uncommon occurrence.

Potential Side Effects of Medicines
Used in the Epidural on the Mother

ANNOYING AND UNPLEASANT SIDE EFFECTS

- Fewer than 10 percent of women report itching all over their body. This disappears as the medication wears off, and medications can be given that are effective in stopping the sensation.
- A common side effect is a drop in blood pressure after the epidural is placed. There are techniques used to try to prevent this from happening, but if your blood pressure decreases it can be quickly brought back to normal by using medications or by changing your position. You may be asked to lie on your side to improve blood flow through the large arteries in your back.
- It is common for women to experience difficulty urinating after an epidural; this sensation disappears when the medication wears off.
- Some women spike a fever, although this is not due to infection (a typical source of fever). It is thought that fever in some women is just their body's response to the epidural itself and usually goes away quickly after giving birth (see the section, "Epidural Concerns and Controversy," page 94, for more information on this potential side effect).
- Shivering after giving birth or during labor is a common side effect after receiving an epidural. If this happens, you will be made more comfortable with warm blankets. Although it is not known why, women who have the shivers with the epidural are more likely to be among the 15 to 20 percent of women who also spike a fever.[5] (Shivering is also often experienced by women who use *no medications* during labor and birth.)
- Nausea is not a common side effect, occurring in less

than 10 percent of women, but when it does occur medications can be given to relieve the queasy feeling.

SERIOUS AND VERY RARE SIDE EFFECTS: A COMMONSENSE PERSPECTIVE ON THE MOST SERIOUS RISKS ASSOCIATED WITH EPIDURALS DURING CHILDBIRTH.

The epidural is a highly safe and effective method used to relieve labor pain by millions of women each year. When considering the issue of safety, it may be helpful to keep in mind that epidurals are used every day *by thousands of patients,* not just laboring women, and grave negative outcomes are extremely rare indeed. The possibility of rare, potentially catastrophic reactions to an epidural are often misstated, or worse, overstated. In fact, most anesthesiologists go through their entire careers without ever seeing a catastrophic outcome as a result of a laboring mother receiving an epidural.

The most serious side effects of the epidural are extraordinarily rare, but extreme consequences can occur if the medication is administered improperly or if the mother has a rare toxic reaction to the medication.

We list below the *extremely rare* negative outcomes of the use of epidurals during childbirth:

- Any time an injection is given to any part of your body, including with an epidural, there is a very rare chance of bleeding or infection.
- A rare toxic reaction to the local anesthetic can cause seizures, paralysis, and death. As indicated in the box on page 90, the chances of anesthesia-related death during childbirth are approximately two in one million.
- If medication is improperly administered or too much is given, the anesthetic medication can reach the chest muscles, which could impact the laboring mother's ability to breathe. In the rare event that this occurs, oxygen is given to the laboring woman. However, if the

problem is undetected, and the anesthetic impairs the
mother's ability to breathe, this could result in death.

Anesthesia-related deaths during childbirth in the United
States have fallen dramatically. In a 1997 report, it was revealed that from 1979 to 1990, maternal deaths related to
anesthesia during childbirth dropped from 4.3 women
per million to 1.7 women per million. This significant
decline, which brings the risk of anesthesia-related death
during childbirth to approximately 2 in a million, is
thought to be due primarily to two factors: (1) the improved safety of regional anesthesia and (2) the increase in
the use of regional anesthesia instead of general anesthesia for cesarean delivery.[6]

Potential Side Effects of the Epidural on the Newborn

The most commonly used method for evaluating the overall
health of a newborn is called the Apgar score. It was named
after an anesthesiologist, Virginia Apgar, who developed this
scoring system in 1953. The Apgar score assesses the baby's
health by evaluating five different variables at one minute, and
then again at five minutes, after birth. A number (score) is assigned to each of the variables and newborns can have an Apgar
score between 1 and 10. The variables measured in the newborn are listed below:

A=Appearance (skin color)
   A score of 0 is given for blue or pale skin color, 1 for
   pink with blue extremities, and 2 for overall pink color.
P=Pulse (heart rate)
   A score of 0 is given for no pulse, 1 for under 100
   beats per minute, and 2 for over 100 beats per minute
   (normal pulse for a healthy newborn ranges from 120
   to 160 beats per minute).

G=Grimace (neurological response)
   A score of 0 is given for nonresponsive grimace, 1 for
   grimace, and 2 for cough or sneeze.
A=Activity (muscle tone)
   A score of 0 is given for limp muscle tone, 1 for
   some reflex, and 2 for active movement.
R=Respiration (breathing)
   A score of 0 is given for no breathing, 1 for slow
   breathing, and 2 for good crying.

Research has consistently shown there is no significant
difference in neonatal outcomes determined by Apgar
scores of babies born to mothers who used an epidural
during labor and birth compared to those who did not.[7]

The medications used in an epidural include a very small
dose of local anesthetic combined with a small amount of a
highly diluted narcotic. Since the epidural medications are
injected into your epidural space (and not into your bloodstream), a small amount of these medications is carried throughout your system, which is why very little of the medication is
passed on to the baby. However, as with all drugs used during
childbirth, *some* amount of medication crosses the placenta and
reaches the baby. It is known that the level of the baby's exposure to the epidural medications during labor is extremely
small.

DID YOU KNOW? *The emergency cesarean delivery for a
distressed baby is* not *more common among women who have
had an epidural.*[8]

• If the drugs in the epidural lower your blood pressure,
   this could result in decreased blood flow to your baby,

slowing down his or her heart rate. This occurs in about 30 percent of laboring women and may be particularly true for those who have had extreme pain and distress prior to receiving the epidural. If this happens, you will be given fluids or, if necessary, you will be treated with medications to bring your own blood pressure back up to normal.

- In very rare cases, a baby of a mother who received an epidural may experience respiratory depression, although this is more likely if the mom has had IV or oral medications during labor.

Epidural Concerns and Controversy: What You May Have Heard Versus What the Research Says

The overwhelming majority of women who receive an epidural have healthy, safe childbirth experiences, free of complications to themselves and their babies. However, many women still feel concerned about the use of an epidural for pain relief during childbirth. Their concerns are often based on inaccurate information about the potential side effects and risks associated with the epidural. In this section we address issues that affect a very small minority of women who experience labor and birth complications, and, as you will see, these complications are often not the result of their choice of pain relief.

EPIDURALS AND CESAREANS—IS THERE REALLY A CONNECTION?

The epidural is often blamed for contributing to the increase in the number of cesarean section births over the last several decades. Some studies suggest an association between the epidural and cesarean births, and other studies conclude that there is no evidence to support such an association. This is probably one of the most hotly debated issues among caregivers concerning the use of epidurals for pain relief during childbirth.

Making the matter even more complicated, there are several

other factors that can influence whether a woman's labor will result in a cesarean delivery, factors such as the woman's age and general health, whether she is giving birth to twins or multiple babies, and the specific cesarean rates of the obstetrician who is attending the birth.

RESEARCH SAYS: *Many researchers believe it is not the use of the epidural that results in a cesarean birth, but the problem that causes the intense pain in the first place. Their research has led them to conclude that labors that are destined to end up with problems, such as failure to progress (dystocia), are inherently more painful right from the beginning, so these women who go on to deliver via cesarean are more likely to request epidurals. One study that supports this theory found that pain during the early stage of labor was directly related to the outcome of labor, and that women who described their pain as horrible or excruciating had three times the cesarean rate as women whose descriptions of their pain were not as severe.*[9]

Researchers at Harvard Medical School who examined the relationship between epidural analgesia and the rate of cesarean delivery found that women who went on to have a cesarean delivery required more pain-relief medication in their epidural during labor than those who went on to give birth vaginally. Their study of over four thousand women who used an epidural for pain relief during labor led these researchers to conclude that "the need for excessive supplemental epidural medication, and perhaps even the request for an epidural, may be markers for severe pain caused by dysfunctional labor."[10]

One method used to determine whether the epidural is responsible for increasing a woman's chance of a cesarean delivery is to compare the cesarean rates of hospitals *before and after* these hospitals offered epidural analgesia as a pain-relief option. In a study that tracked over thirty-seven thousand births in hospitals in several different countries over a period of many years, it was shown that increasing the use of epidural analgesia in hospitals from very low levels to very high usage (sometimes as much as a five- to tenfold increase) *did not increase* the rate of cesarean delivery.[11]

The authors of one study suggested that if epidural analgesia was a key factor in determining rising cesarean section rates, obstetricians who used epidurals more frequently with their patients during labor would have higher rates of cesarean sections. Their study followed 110 obstetricians caring for approximately fifty low-risk moms each. They concluded: "The frequency of use of epidural analgesia does not predict obstetricians' rates of cesarean section for dystocia. After accounting for a number of known patient risk factors, obstetrical practice style appears to be a major determinant of rates of cesarean section."[12]

In a more neutral stance on this issue, one review that involved over three thousand women set out to explore the potential negative effects of the epidural compared to nonepidural pain relief, including no pain-relief intervention at all. Regarding the specific issue of the epidural and its possible association with cesarean deliveries, this review concluded: "No statistically significant effect on cesarean section rates could be identified. Epidural analgesia appears to be very effective in reducing pain during labor, although there appear to be some potentially adverse effects. Further research is needed to investigate adverse effects and to evaluate the different techniques used in epidural analgesia."[13]

WILL YOUR CHANCES OF SPIKING A FEVER INCREASE WITH AN EPIDURAL?

Yes, there is a known connection between the use of epidural analgesia and an increase in the number of women who spike a fever during or after labor. The most recent research shows that elevated temperature associated with the epidural occurs in 24 percent of women having their first baby.[14] It is thought that fever associated with an epidural may have something to do with a long labor. Fever among repeat moms who use an epidural is far less common, possibly due to the fact that this group typically spends less time in labor than first-time moms.

RESEARCH SAYS: *One theory regarding the cause of a laboring woman's fever after an epidural is that during painful labor women breathe very fast, which allows heat to dissipate from their body, keeping them cool. Women who are using an epidural tend to have calm and relaxed breathing patterns, which may actually result in a rise in temperature. The fever itself rarely causes a problem in the mother or baby; the newborn, however, is more likely to be seen for a "sepsis workup" to make certain he or she does not have an infection. Previously, this was done by giving the baby a spinal tap, using a needle to extract spinal fluid. This procedure is almost never used these days, and a simple blood test is all that is needed to determine the baby's health status. Babies born to mothers who have had an epidural may also be more likely to receive precautionary antibiotics; studies have shown, however, that the rate of infection among these babies is not higher than the rate of infection among babies born to mothers who did not use an epidural.[15]*

DO EPIDURALS CAUSE LOWER BACK PAIN?

Once an epidural is removed, some women have localized back pain at the site where the epidural needle was inserted. This tenderness should last only a day or two. Many women describe feeling generalized lower back pain after an epidural, and others have reported continued back pain for months or even years after the birth of their baby.

Often the epidural is thought of as the culprit for these lower-back ailments, but mothers who have given birth naturally, without the use of an epidural, *also* experience generalized lower back pain after birth, sometimes for months or even years after the birth of their baby. There is no known connection between the use of an epidural during childbirth and future lower-back problems.

RESEARCH SAYS: *A recent study to determine whether the use of an epidural during labor is associated with long-term backache, followed 369 women and concluded: "After childbirth there are no differences in the incidence of long-term low back pain, disability, or movement restriction between women who receive epidural pain relief and women who receive other forms of pain relief."*[16]

WHAT *DOES* CAUSE THIS LOWER BACK PAIN?

Researchers aren't exactly sure, but it is known that during pregnancy, hormonal changes cause the ligaments in your body to soften. This, combined with the extra weight carried during pregnancy, can put increased strain on your lower back, which can result in back pain that may continue well after childbirth.

Unfortunately, once you give birth, the strain on your lower back does not decrease: you are now carrying around a growing bundle of joy, lifting car seats and strollers, and schlepping well-stocked diaper bags throughout your day. It has been suggested that lower back pain often accompanies the job of mothering infants and toddlers and that the form of pain relief used during labor and birth is unrelated to this condition.

DOES THE EPIDURAL LENGTHEN LABOR?

It is known that in some women, an epidural can slow down labor, in particular the second stage of labor, by about twenty-five minutes to an hour. It is not known exactly why this is so; many women, however, are willing to take the chance of tacking on more time of pain-free labor rather than experiencing a slightly shorter, but more painful, labor and delivery.

> **RESEARCH SAYS:** *In a recent study that examined the birth outcomes of over two thousand first-time moms, approximately half of whom received an epidural and half used narcotic pain relief, it was observed that the moms who used an epidural during labor had longer first and second stages of labor.*[17]

DOES THE EPIDURAL INCREASE YOUR CHANCES OF HAVING AN ASSISTED DELIVERY?

The use of forceps (a device used by the obstetrician to assist the baby down the birth canal) is associated with a higher rate of laceration (tears) to the mom's vagina and rectal area. There is an association with the use of the epidural and the increased use of forceps or vacuum extraction (a suction device used by the obstetrician to assist the baby down the birth canal) during childbirth; the nature of this association, however, is unclear.

Forceps and vacuum extraction during delivery are used when the baby is stuck in the birth canal, often due to the fact that it is not in the proper birthing position. It is not known whether the effects of the epidural on the uterine muscles prevent the baby from turning itself into the proper birthing position, or if the baby starts out in the wrong position, causing severe pain to the mother, who then requests an epidural.

The use of forceps during birth, whether or not women use an epidural, is highly dependent on many factors, including your individual obstetrician's practice style.[18] Some obstetricians use instruments more frequently during childbirth than others. In addition, there is variation among obstetricians with regard to how they use the instruments. Some obstetricians are very gentle and skilled at using forceps, with minimal discomfort or tearing to the mother and baby, and others may be less so. The research on this aspect of the use of epidurals is conflicting, with some studies showing an association and others suggesting there is none.

Newer forms of the epidural, such as the combined spinal epidural (CSE) and patient-controlled epidural analgesia (PCEA), which use lower doses of medications (see page 101–115), allow for more sensation during the pushing stage but can still provide adequate pain relief and make it easier for women to push, possibly making the need for forceps less likely.

> **RESEARCH SAYS:** *One study that compared the low-dose epidural with the conventional epidural in over one thousand first-time moms found that the women who used the lower-dose form of epidural (combined spinal epidural), versus the conventional epidural, had over a 7 percent increase in normal vaginal delivery rate. The study concluded: "The use of low-dose epidural techniques for labor analgesia has benefits for the delivery outcome."*[19]

The most recent studies comparing epidurals to IV narcotic pain relief found an *increase* in the rate of deliveries involving forceps from 7 percent in the IV and oral medication (narcotics) group to 13 percent in the group of women who used epidural analgesia. The study concluded, however, that "epidural analgesia compared to intravenous analgesia (meperidine) during labor does *not* increase the number of *cesarean deliveries.*"[20]

A separate study—which compared the rate of instrument-assisted births in a hospital where only 1 percent of women used epidural analgesia, to the rate one year later, when the hospital, in that twelve-month period, increased its epidural usage rate to 84 percent of women, while all other conditions remained unchanged—concluded: "Overall instrumental delivery did not increase. Epidural analgesia during labor does not increase the risk of cesarean delivery, nor does it necessarily increase oxytocin use, or instrumental delivery caused by dystocia."[21]

But I'm Parched! Oral Intake with an Epidural

The restriction of food and drink during labor is still a widely practiced policy in hospital labor and delivery units. The reason women have been restricted from eating or drinking during labor has to do with reducing the risk of inhaling vomited material into your lungs if, in the event of an emergency, you must receive general anesthesia. Although this rarely occurs, it can put the woman at risk for pneumonia. In extremely rare cases, it can result in death due to failed emergency attempts to clear the laboring woman's airway.

Many hospitals are now beginning to allow women clear liquid intake during labor, which means they may have some types of juices, tea, clear broth, popsicles, or Jell-O. Local hospital practices will differ, so check with your own hospital for details on its oral-intake policy on the maternity unit.

> **RESEARCH SAYS:** *Recent evidence indicates* no change in amount of vomiting *in a group of women allowed to drink sports drinks, such as Gatorade, during labor versus those who were restricted to only ice chips. And we can guess which group was* more satisfied *with its choice of hydration.*[22]

As a precaution, certain patients, especially those who are at greatest risk for cesarean section, may still be subject to more restrictive fluid-intake policies. Women who are scheduled for an elective cesarean are always asked to restrict food and liquid completely for at least six to eight hours before surgery.

The Epidural and Your Baby's Breast-Feeding Success

Controversy has recently surfaced over whether the use of an epidural during labor has an impact on overall success rates for breast-feeding. Some women may experience difficulty with breast-feeding for a variety of reasons, regardless of the method of anesthesia, or whether they use pain-relief medications at all during labor. The examination of breast milk of women who used epidurals indicates that the amount of medications (anesthetics and narcotics) found in the milk is very low, even after prolonged epidural infusions.

The use of an epidural for pain relief during labor does not adversely impact the baby's or mother's ability to breast-feed. It appears that the most important factor regarding the success of breast-feeding is support for a mother's breast-feeding efforts through extensive caregiver support and teaching, and early contact between mother and newborn.

RESEARCH SAYS: *Researchers asked 171 healthy women who had given birth six weeks earlier to describe their breast-feeding status, including problems encountered, solutions found, sources of support and information, and their sense of satisfaction. Sixty percent of these women used an epidural for pain relief during labor. Of these women, 72 percent breast-fed fully and 20 percent breast-fed partially. The authors stated: "We could not demonstrate a correlation between breast-feeding success at 6 to 8 weeks and epidural analgesia. In a hospital that strongly promotes breast-feeding, epidural analgesia with local anesthetics and opioids does not impede breast-feeding success. We recommend that hospitals that find decreased (breast-feeding) success in mothers receiving an epidural reexamine their post-delivery care policies."*[23]

In addition, a recent Italian study, which followed nineteen hundred women after they gave birth vaginally, found that there was no difference in the number of women who were breast-feeding their infants at the time of their discharge from the hospital, regardless of whether these women *did* or *did not* use an epidural during labor.[24]

The Combined Spinal Epidural (CSE)

> **Did You Know?** *The combined spinal epidural (CSE) is quickly becoming a popular technique for treating labor pain. An increasing number of hospitals are now offering the CSE as a pain-relief option in addition to the option of the conventional epidural.*

What It Is and What It Does
The combination of both spinal and epidural methods for pain relief is sometimes called the walking epidural or epidural–lite and was created to enhance women's satisfaction with their childbirth experience.

The CSE uses both the spinal *and* epidural methods of pain relief combined in one procedure, to achieve pain relief during childbirth. The spinal injection offers rapid, almost instant pain relief, usually within two or three contractions, and the epidural provides ongoing pain relief throughout the rest of labor and birth, or for as long as you may need it. The CSE is designed to give you enough pain relief to make you comfortable while allowing you some mobility to reposition yourself in bed, move from bed to chair, or possibly to walk (with assistance) during labor.

How It's Done and How It Feels
The procedure for the CSE is the same as the basic epidural placement (see page 77), except that in the CSE, there is *one additional step:* once the epidural needle is in place, a thin spinal needle is inserted through the epidural needle and an injection of medication is given directly into the sac of fluid containing your nerves and spinal cord. Since the spinal needle is placed through the inside of the epidural needle, it does *not* require an additional puncture in your back and will not cause you any pain.

Medications Used in the CSE

The types of medications used in the CSE are the same as those used in a conventional epidural—a narcotic and a local anesthetic—but the *amount* of medication given is less. Even though a smaller amount of medication is used, its effect is rapid and highly effective because it is injected directly into the spinal space, where the nerves are located—unlike the epidural, in which the medication is injected just outside of the spinal space.

When Can You Get a CSE?

The timing considerations for a CSE are the same as for an epidural; the increased use of the CSE, however, has made a big impact on the willingness of anesthesiologists to give an epidural late in labor. How this issue is dealt with can vary among different hospitals and physicians.

What You May Feel When the CSE Starts to Work

You will feel more comfortable, with little or no pain, after receiving a CSE. You may still feel your contractions, but the pain will be significantly diminished or entirely eliminated by the medications. You will not feel the sensation of complete numbness from the chest down, which you might feel with a conventional epidural. Since the CSE uses less medication, you will still be able to move your legs; in some cases, you may be able to sit up comfortably, or even walk around with assistance.

The medications given in the spinal part of the CSE begin to wear off after around ninety minutes. If you are still in labor and need pain relief, medications can be added to the epidural to keep you comfortable.

DID YOU KNOW? *Women who use the CSE for pain relief during childbirth have higher patient satisfaction than women who use a standard epidural.*[25]

What Your Partner Can Do

Just as with an epidural, the fact that your pain has gone does not mean that your partner no longer plays an important role. In fact, now that you are feeling comfortable, your partner may be better able to help you reposition in bed, or assist you in getting out of bed and support you while you move around.

Reasons You May Choose the CSE

- The CSE offers almost instant pain relief.
- You want the advantage of more mobility during labor.
- You want to reduce pain but do not want to experience complete numbness during labor and birth.

Potential Side Effects of the CSE

The potential side effects of the CSE are the same as those for the conventional epidural (see pages 88–92), and may include a drop in blood pressure; itchiness, especially on the face; and nausea and vomiting. All of these symptoms can be reduced or prevented with medication.

Potential Benefits of the CSE

- The CSE works especially well to provide rapid relief to women in *early labor* (two to three centimeters dilated) whose labor pain has not been relieved by other methods.
- The CSE is especially advantageous for women who need pain relief *late in labor,* since it can eliminate pain so quickly and does not affect the ability to move your legs and push out the baby.
- Overall, with a CSE, as compared to an epidural, a much smaller amount of medication is used, so less will reach your baby's system.
- Women who want to avoid IV medications or sedatives may prefer the CSE.
- If you are in need of an emergency cesarean section, the

epidural part of the CSE will provide anesthesia throughout the surgery.
- The epidural part of the CSE allows for your medications to
continue for as long as you need pain relief. The medication
dosages may be increased if your labor intensifies.
- With the CSE you may have increased effectiveness
(compared to the epidural) during the pushing stage, since
you are not completely without sensation. You may find it
easier to shift, turn, or squat during labor and delivery.

Potential Limitations of the CSE

- Although you are more mobile than with a conventional
epidural, you may not be able to actually *walk* around, for
a number of reasons. You may not have the strength in
your legs, or you may simply not feel well enough at this
point in your labor to walk around, or your hospital may
have policies that prevent you from walking around, for
liability reasons.

Conditions That May Prevent You from Getting a CSE

- You have a history of blood clotting or take certain
medications that can affect blood clotting. You should
discuss all of this with your obstetrician or an
anesthesiologist prior to going into labor.
- You have certain neurological disorders.
- You have previously had certain lower-back surgical
procedures.
- During childbirth you prefer to avoid the use of anything
more high-tech than the massage setting on your
showerhead.

About 5 percent of the time, the physician cannot get the spinal
needle into the exact location needed to administer the medications, even though the epidural needle is placed perfectly. If
this happens, the epidural is used for pain relief.

RESEARCH SAYS: *One study of 1,532 healthy laboring women cited these results: "Anesthesiologists were more likely to use the CSE than the epidural for repeat moms than for first-time moms. The CSE was used more in women who were having more painful labor and who were toward the end of their labor. The side effect of itching occurred more in women who used the CSE than in women who used an epidural." There was no difference in the method of delivery (vaginal or cesarean) detected between the two groups.*[26]

A review of over two thousand women who used the CSE during labor concluded: "Compared with the epidural, the CSE provides faster onset of effective pain relief from the time of injection, and increases the incidence of maternal satisfaction. However, CSE women experience more itch. There is no difference between CSE and epidural techniques with respect to: the incidence of forceps delivery, maternal mobility, headache due to post dural puncture, cesarean section rates or admission of babies to the neonatal unit."[27]

THE PATIENT-CONTROLLED EPIDURAL ANALGESIA (PCEA)

DID YOU KNOW? *This form of pain relief is growing in usage and popularity throughout the United States. Studies show that laboring women use less analgesic medication for pain relief when they can administer their own dosage.*

What It Is and What It Does

If an epidural is the Cadillac of all medical pain-relief options, the patient-controlled epidural analgesia (PCEA) is the pain-relief option that gives *you* the steering wheel. The PCEA is an epidural connected to a special pump that is programmed by your anesthesiologist to release the amount of medication necessary for pain relief throughout your labor and birth. You are given a handheld control that operates the pump; by pressing the button on the control you are able to release the amount of medication needed to keep you comfortable. The primary advantage of this type of epidural is that *you* have control over how much medication is given, and you can adjust this based on how uncomfortable your labor feels.

Studies have shown that there is often a reduction in the amount of medication used when women control delivery of their own medication as compared to women who receive a conventional epidural.

> Don't worry about accidentally giving yourself too much medication. The amount of medication you may give yourself is *not* unlimited. In fact, you are only able to give yourself the preallotted medicine in doses measured by your anesthesiologist. A precise timing mechanism, called a lockout device, prevents the possibility of overdosing.

Often the PCEA will also run a small amount of continuous pain-relief medication, which helps maintain your comfort level by keeping the flow of medication consistent. The PCEA, like the conventional epidural, reduces or eliminates painful sensations during labor. Typically the PCEA is given in lower doses than a traditional epidural, but the pain relief is extremely effective and can keep women pain-free, or nearly pain-free, throughout labor and birth. Once it is in place, the PCEA begins working within fifteen to twenty minutes.

How It's Done and How It Feels
The PCEA is administered by the anesthesiologist exactly like an epidural (see page 77). In addition, when the laboring mom is ready for the PCEA to be placed, the anesthesiologist or

nurse teaches the patient and her support person how the PCEA works and shows her how to comfortably operate the pump on her own.

HEY, THERE'S SOME LEFT OVER.
(CAN WE TAKE THIS "TO GO"?)

Women who use the PCEA often do not need as much pain-relief medicine as women who are given a traditional epidural. One recent study showed that, *even when ultra-low doses of medications were used,* women who used the PCEA did not give themselves as much pain-relief medication as is typically used in an epidural.[28]

How You May Feel Once Your PCEA Is in Place
Some women find that they have a satisfying sense of control over their birth experience by managing their own comfort level. Others report feeling concerned about their own ability to give themselves enough medication to keep them comfortable, and others worry that they will use too much pain medication. Your nurses and your anesthesiologist will check with you often to be sure the dosage you are giving yourself is effectively relieving your pain. Typically, as labor progresses, the pain becomes more severe; therefore the best pain-management approach is to continue giving yourself as much medication as needed to stay comfortable rather than trying to conserve on your pain medication. If you attempt to cut back on the medication and your labor intensifies, it can be difficult to catch up with the pain as it becomes more severe.

Just as with an epidural, you and your baby will be monitored from this point on, until your baby's birth. You will wear two belts around your belly, the electronic fetal monitor, which monitors the baby, and the tocodynamometer, which measures your contractions. The PCEA can stay in for as long as you need pain relief, including throughout the initial part of your recovery, until you and your doctor determine you are ready to discontinue the pain-relief medications, or your doctor switches you to oral pain relievers. The removal of the PCEA catheter from your back is completely painless.

Medications Used in the PCEA
The medications used are the same as in an epidural—typically a small amount of a local anesthetic and a narcotic—but they are given in smaller doses.

When Can You Get a PCEA?
Since the PCEA is basically an epidural, the issues around timing are the same. The PCEA can be started at almost any point during the first stage of labor.

Potential Benefits of the PCEA Versus the Epidural and Other Types of Pain Relief

- The psychological and emotional benefit of feeling a sense of control during childbirth can increase your satisfaction with your birth experience.
- Many women end up using less medication with a PCEA compared to a conventional epidural.
- You have instant control over obtaining additional pain relief when needed, rather than waiting for the anesthesiologist to provide you with another dose of medicine.
- The PCEA is the only method of pain relief in which the amount of medication is tailored specifically to address the amount of pain you are experiencing by adjusting the pump to increase or decrease medication. This can help you avoid overtreating or undertreating your pain.
- The PCEA usually provides greater mobility and often allows women to walk around, with assistance.
- The pain relief provided is fast and highly effective, and works within fifteen to twenty minutes.

Potential Limitation of Using the PCEA

• The most conspicuous limitation is that not all hospitals offer PCEA on their labor and delivery units.

Potential Side Effects of the PCEA

• The potential side effects of the PCEA are the same as for the traditional epidural (see pages 88–92).

What Your Partner Can Do

Your partner can help by making sure you are comfortable using the pump and can attend to any other needs you may have now that your pain is diminished. But, the pump is for your use only—no matter how much your partner may love gadgets, he will *not* be allowed to operate the device.

Although this is a fairly new method of pain relief for women during childbirth, much research has been conducted on the PCEA, and its safety is well established.

> **RESEARCH SAYS:** *One recent study concluded: "Patient Controlled Epidural Analgesia [patients] were less likely to need unscheduled anesthetic interventions [from the physician], they receive a slightly lower dose of local anesthetic, and have less motor block [numbness] than those who have continuous epidural infusion."*[29]

The Five Key Questions You Should Ask About Anesthesia Coverage at Your Hospital

Anesthesia during childbirth is one of the most important considerations of your labor. If you plan to opt for medical relief, or even if you are unsure, it is essential that, prior to your delivery, you discuss the various pain-relief options that may or may not be available to you. Here are some of the questions you should ask an anesthesiologist at the hospital where you plan to have your baby:

1. Is an anesthesiologist or nurse-anesthetist *specifically* assigned to the labor and delivery unit, or is he or she responsible for coverage of the *entire* hospital?
2. What types of epidurals are available on the labor and delivery unit? Do you offer CSEs or PCEAs?
3. Does my doctor (or hospital) have a policy or practice guideline regarding when an epidural can be given? What is it and is there any flexibility depending upon patient request?
4. Is the anesthesiologist *in the hospital around the clock* or does he or she take calls from home?—There is often a difference in how quickly you may be attended to, based on the answer to this question. The anesthesiologist who is available "on call," around the clock, but is not physically in the hospital when you need him or her, will most likely not be as readily available to you as the anesthesiologist who is available in the hospital twenty-four hours a day, seven days a week.
5. Can I meet with someone in the anesthesiology department before I arrive at the labor and delivery unit?—This may or may not be part of your childbirth preparation, so you may need to take your own initiative if your hospital does not routinely offer a time to meet with the anesthesiology department.

A Caregiver's Perspective on the PCEA

Holly Muir, M.D., chief of women's anesthesiology, Duke University Health System, Durham, North Carolina

"I have been using the PCEA since 1992. Women really like the ability to have some control over their own pain management during childbirth. Most women come in knowing that they can request the 'epidural with a button,' which they have learned in their childbirth preparation course will be made available to them on the birthing unit.

"The nursing staff likes that the PCEA empowers laboring women by giving them more control over this aspect of their childbirth. Patients can choose the timing of the PCEA in our hospital. When they feel their pain is such that they need relief, the anesthesiologist administers the PCEA and provides instruction on its use."

What Women Say About Epidurals

Laura Chritton, a mother of two who had a doula and an epidural with her first baby, and had an epidural with her second baby

Why Did You Decide to Use an Epidural?

"For my first baby, I had the support of a doula and had hoped to have a natural childbirth. I used breathing techniques to manage the pain. I am an opera singer, so I understand the importance of breathing properly (also, I had been taking yoga). But the breathing techniques did not help me with the pain, and finally, after a very long and painful labor, I requested an epidural. In retrospect, I think I felt I needed to prove something to myself and my doula—that I could give birth naturally."

How Was Your Partner Involved?

"My husband was my masseur! He was very supportive of my having a natural birth, but once I decided on the epidural he was also fine with that decision. My husband is an anesthesiologist, but not on the labor and delivery unit!"

Would You Use an Epidural Again? Would You Recommend It to Other Women?

"Yes, I used an epidural for my second baby. The second time around I didn't feel as if I needed to see how much pain I could endure; all I wanted was a healthy baby. The second time I went straight to an epidural; it was 'Just give me the drugs!'

The epidural allowed me to be present during the birth. I was assured I would feel pressure, not pain, and that is exactly what happened. I felt every contraction and let everyone know when I felt ready to push. I think women need to decide for themselves whether they should use the epidural for pain relief, based on their own desires."

Do You Think the Relief of Your Pain Impacted Your Satisfaction with Your Birth?

"Yes, for my first birth especially, less pain would have been better. I wish I had taken pain relief earlier during my first childbirth."

Jennifer Cron, a mother of one who chose to use an epidural during labor

Why Did You Decide to Use an Epidural?

"I wanted to have as little pain as possible in order to have a more pleasant birthing experience."

Was It What You Expected?

"I didn't realize there would still be so much discomfort during pushing. It did provide pain relief for the contractions. Once I got the epidural, I didn't feel any pain until I began pushing. Since the doctor turned down the medication just before I was ready to push, my pain relief wore off, and pushing was painful."

Did You Use Any Other Comfort Measures or Pain-Relief Interventions?

"No."

Do You Think the Relief of Your Pain Impacted Your Satisfaction with Your Birth?

"I do think that my pain relief helped me to have a more satisfying birth experience. I don't really think that I could have experienced less pain, but I do think that if I had experienced more pain, it would have been more of a *trauma* than a satisfying birth experience."

Elizabeth, a mother of two who used an epidural with both births

Why Did You Decide to Use an Epidural?
"I used an epidural for pain management. I was very afraid of the pain of childbirth."

Was It What You Expected?
"I'm not sure what I expected. I was pretty nervous. With the first delivery, I had some complications and ended up having a forceps delivery. The epidural was a godsend. I didn't feel any pain *during* the delivery. My second delivery was a different story. The epidural only affected half of my body, which I knew sometimes happens. When the anesthesiologist 'fixed' it, I ended up unable to feel half of my body at all. It felt like a sandbag and the other half of my body felt everything. It made it very difficult and painful to push. The anesthesiologist was unable to come back to me because he was busy with other patients. It was not a good experience."

How Was Your Partner Involved?
"He helped me with the breathing and to stay focused. He was very supportive and gave me a lot of positive feedback like, 'You're doing great,' and that kind of thing. I am very glad he was there with me."

Would You Use the Epidural Again? Would
You Recommend It to Other Women?
"I would recommend learning the breathing exercises. [If nothing else, they give you something to focus on.] And I would recommend getting an epidural as soon as possible."

*Do You Think the Relief of Your Pain Impacted
Your Satisfaction with Your Birth?*

"I think to some degree the satisfaction with your birth experience is out of your control. I felt more satisfied with my
second birth experience because I actually pushed my daughter
out (my first birth experience was a forceps delivery). But, I
think to some degree, the less pain you feel, the more satisfying
the experience. I would also say that I would not want to be
doped up on something that makes you so out of it that you
don't remember the experience or are not yourself."

Amy Siverd, a mother of one and expecting another

Why Did You Decide to Use an Epidural?

"I was sick with preeclampsia and had to be induced. We
began ripening my cervix the night before since it was fully
closed. I woke up in the middle of the night in severe pain. I
was given Demerol and this took the edge off and allowed me
to sleep some more before the induction. We began Pitocin
when I was one centimeter dilated. By the time I was five centimeters dilated, I was having breathtaking contractions that
were nonstop. I begged for the epidural at that point. I couldn't
imagine having to continue without it."

Did the Epidural Provide Pain Relief?

"It was amazing how much better I felt. The epidural was
better than I expected. I feel fortunate to have had the option.
I still felt the tightening of my uterus but the intense, nauseat-
ing pain was gone. I felt great after labor and did not need any
more pain relief."

How Was Your Partner Involved?

"He was absolutely not involved—this was *my* pain. He
just felt helpless. It was a relief for both of us when the pain
was managed. We were able to concentrate on the delivery,
finally."

Would You Use the Epidural Again? Would You Recommend It to Other Women?

"I will absolutely use an epidural again. I just hope I get it sooner. As far as recommending an epidural to others, probably not. Pain relief is a personal choice that is best made by educating yourself about all pain-relief options. Just because I had a great experience doesn't mean someone else will. I'm happy I made the decision to get an epidural, but I don't necessarily need to wear the T-shirt!"

Five

EASING THE PAIN

Medications to Relieve
(But Not Eliminate) Your Pain

Pain medications have been used for centuries to ease the pain of childbirth. Modern pain-relief medication may provide adequate pain control for some women, but generally speaking, women who seek to reduce the pain of labor and birth should be aware that other pain medications are not as effective in providing relief as are all forms of the epidural. Compared to the epidural, medications given intravenously or by injection carry different risks to both mother and baby, and they often cause unpleasant side effects. Women who prefer not to have an epidural may, however, find that a well-timed injection of a pain reliever can make all the difference in coping with their labor pain, allowing them to achieve their goal of avoiding the use of an epidural.

How these medications may impact you and your newborn will depend on the type of drug used, how much is given, and when you receive the medication. The effect on the baby is typically more apparent when the medications are given close to the time of birth, since they have not had time to be metabolized by the newborn.

In this chapter we discuss:

- The most common modern pain-relief medications used during childbirth.
- The patient-controlled analgesia (pain relief) pump.
- The pudendal block for pain relief.
- The use of nitrous oxide, wildly popular in Britain, but less so in the United States.

PAIN-RELIEF MEDICATIONS

The epidural is the most effective form of medical pain relief used during childbirth, but not everyone who is comfortable using pain-relief medications prefers the epidural.

> **DID YOU KNOW?** *Parenteral narcotics (medications given intravenously or via injection) are used by 39 to 56 percent of women in labor in U.S. hospitals. Many of the women who use pain-relief medications also go on to request an epidural.*[1]

Reasons You May Choose Pain-Relief Medications During Labor

- You are trying *not* to use medical pain relief but your labor is more painful than you had anticipated (or your caregivers indicated) and you need a little help in taking the edge off.
- You plan to have an epidural but you are not able to receive one immediately.
- You want to avoid the use of an epidural for pain relief but want the benefits of modern medicine during your childbirth experience.
- You need temporary relief from your pain to rest and conserve your energy for active labor.
- For medical reasons you are unable to have an epidural.

Reasons You May Not Choose Pain-Relief Medications During Labor

- You simply prefer not to take any medications and have prepared yourself to cope with the rigors of labor by using another method of pain management.
- It is your desire to remain fully alert, not groggy or sleepy, during your childbirth.

PAIN-RELIEF MEDICATIONS VERSUS THE EPIDURAL

Studies have shown that, compared with the epidural, pain-relief medications given intravenously or through injections are not only *less effective* in providing pain relief but also have *lower patient satisfaction* regarding pain relief in all stages of labor, often as a result of the medications' unpleasant side effects.[2]

Pain-relief medications used during childbirth can be given in a few different ways, depending on the type of medication itself, your own preference, and the capacity of the hospital or birth center where you decide to give birth. Typically, pain-relief medications on the labor unit are ordered by the obstetrician, anesthesiologist, or midwife, and are given to you by the nurses or midwife.

Most often, pain-relief medications are given through an IV that is inserted into a vein on the back of your hand or your arm. Unless you prefer otherwise, an IV is usually placed routinely in laboring women to help keep you hydrated during labor. The advantage of an IV over injections is that you will only need one needle stick, since the medications can be administered through the IV bag or tube rather than given through additional injections. The disadvantage is that you are now connected to an IV tube and pole, and if you feel like staying mobile during your labor, this apparatus will need to move with you. If you do not want an IV, many of the pain-relief medications used can also be given through an injection into a muscle in your arm, thigh, or buttocks and then given again if and when more pain relief is needed. If you prefer a shot over the insertion of an IV, this is a simple way to receive your medication, but the pain-relief effects do not kick in as quickly. Be sure to check with your own hospital about its IV policy for women during labor.

> **DID YOU KNOW?** *Pain-relief medications given by injection can take up to forty-five minutes to take full effect. Pain-relief medications given through an IV typically take around five minutes before you begin to experience relief.*

Some hospitals offer the use of a patient-controlled analgesia (PCA) pump, which is an IV pump with a control button that allows *you* to deliver *your own* dose of medications. The PCA has been used in the hospital setting for over forty years but has only recently gained popularity on the maternity unit. Similar to the patient-controlled epidural analgesia (PCEA) pump, this type of pain-relief device gives you the ability to control how much medication you would like to receive and when you would like to receive it. The pump is preprogrammed with a specific amount of medication(s) and has a safety measure built in that prevents you from accidentally overdosing.

What Your Partner Can Do When You Are Using Pain-Relief Medications

- Continue to provide emotional support to you during labor.
- Help you get up and around, or at least in and out of the bathroom as needed.

- Encourage you as you approach the next phase of labor.
- Provide physical touch, massage, or stroking for as long as you find it soothing.

While you are resting, your partner should also take time to rest—you will *both* need lots of energy for the next phase of labor.

You will *not* become addicted to narcotics by using them during childbirth.

MODERN PAIN MEDICATIONS FOR CHILDBIRTH

The type of medication, the amount given to women, and the manner in which women receive these medications varies depending on the birth setting, your preferences, and the preferences of your caregivers. There are several different types of drugs used to relieve pain, and the similarities among these medications far outweigh the minor differences. These drugs, called narcotics, all work to relieve pain by the same mechanism: they act by stimulating pain-relieving receptors in the brain and spinal cord. The effectiveness of pain-relief medications (and the side effects they may produce) is mostly dependent on the *amount* of medication given rather than the *type* of medication used.[3]

How each individual laboring woman responds to these medications can vary. Many women experience side effects; others experience none. The amount of pain relief experienced can also differ among women. Some women report that their pain is greatly diminished by medications, whereas other women continue to experience significant pain in spite of the use of pain-relief medications.

> ### Your Options Are Still Open
>
> Many of these medications can be used during early labor, even if you decide to opt for an epidural later in your labor.

The Most Common *Types* of Medications Used During Childbirth

Unless you have dreams of becoming a pharmacist, you are probably not going to memorize the names and characteristics of every medication available to you in the delivery room. So, in order to keep the process of learning about pain-relief medications pain-free, we will list the medications most *commonly* used during childbirth and provide straightforward information on how they may impact you and your newborn.

To start, there are different types of pain-relief medications available once you go into labor. Sedatives will provide relaxation, but will not relieve your pain. Analgesics or narcotics (pain relievers) will help to "take the edge off" your pain, and local anesthetics will numb the site on the body where the medication is injected (similar to the numbing shot you may receive at your dentist's office).

Sedatives
Sedatives are medications that induce relaxation and cause drowsiness. These are not pain relievers but are used to help decrease your anxiety if you are especially tense or anxious at the start of labor. Sedatives also help promote rest or sleep. Drugs in this category affect the entire nervous system and take effect over your whole body (systemic) instead of affecting one particular area. The sedative effect of most of the medications used during labor peaks about an hour after receiving the medi-

cation if given by pill, and at around thirty minutes if given via injection.

WHEN CAN YOU GET THEM?

Sedatives are most commonly given at the beginning of labor, if you are experiencing anxiety or are unable to rest. Your physician may even send you home with a sedative that will permit you to rest or sleep until your labor increases and you are ready to return to the maternity unit.

THE POTENTIAL BENEFIT OF SEDATIVES DURING CHILDBIRTH

These medications promote rest and may provide relief by reducing your anxiety level and, in doing so, can significantly add to your sense of comfort and well-being during this early stage of labor.

WHAT YOU MAY FEEL WHEN GIVEN A SEDATIVE DURING LABOR

A sedative will most likely make you feel sleepy, relaxed, and possibly light-headed or "floaty." It is possible that you will sleep for a short time, or rest more comfortably if needed. Since the ideal is to remain active for as long as possible, especially in early labor, women are not typically given a sedative unless they report a significant amount of anxiety or have been awake, with no rest, for several hours, in uncomfortable or painful early labor. The rest provided by a sedative does not necessarily prevent you from actively participating later, as your labor progresses. In fact, the rest gained as a result of the sedative may give you the energy needed to get you back on track for the remainder of your childbirth.

MOST COMMONLY USED SEDATIVES DURING CHILDBIRTH

Seconal (Secobarbital)

This is a medication whose effects do not last long and that promotes relaxation and rest. This medication is typically taken orally, in pill form, or given via injection.

Valium (Diazepam)

This produces an effect similar to that of Seconal. This medication does not provide pain relief but does help reduce anxiety, and may produce a moderate amnesia-like effect in some women.

THE POTENTIAL SIDE EFFECTS OF SEDATIVES

On You

You may experience any (or none) of the following side effects: dizziness, nausea, vomiting, sleepiness, and a slowed heart rate.

On Your Baby

When a single dose of a sedative is given to women early in labor, there is only a rare chance that the newborn will experience side effects due to the medication. The chances of the newborn experiencing side effects due to the mom's use of sedatives increase, however, if the baby is delivered soon after the mom receives the medication. The risk of the baby becoming sleepy as a result of the mom's use of sedatives also increases when the sedative is given via IV or injection, in combination with a narcotic. The main problem with a sleepy baby is that his or her heart rate and breathing slow. In addition, some babies who have been exposed to sedatives before birth may have difficulty initiating breast-feeding after delivery, and some may have difficulty maintaining a normal body temperature.

Analgesics

Analgesics are pain-reducing medications, also known as narcotics or opioids, and are derived from the poppy plant. These medications can help reduce the intensity of your pain, but they do not affect the intensity of your contractions. Analgesics easily cross the placenta into the baby's bloodstream.

WHEN CAN YOU GET THEM?

If you are having a difficult early labor, you may be given an analgesic in combination with a sedative to help relieve your pain and promote relaxation before active labor begins. Most women do not receive more than a dose or two before getting an epidural.

THE POTENTIAL BENEFITS OF ANALGESICS DURING LABOR

Although narcotics used during labor will most likely not eliminate all of your pain, these medications can make a significant difference in your comfort level. If you are trying to avoid an epidural or cannot have an epidural, the use of narcotics during labor can help reduce your pain from early labor all the way to the birth of your baby.

WHAT YOU MAY FEEL WHEN GIVEN AN ANALGESIC DURING LABOR

You should feel a significant reduction in the intensity of the pain that comes with each contraction. This will feel like a relief for many women. You may also feel groggy, light-headed, or dreamlike. Some women report feeling blissful and euphoric. Others experience the sensation as a loss of control and do not like feeling a lack of clarity during their childbirth, even though their pain may be effectively diminished.

MOST COMMONLY USED ANALGESICS
DURING CHILDBIRTH

Demerol (Also Known as Meperidine—in Britain and Some Other Countries It Is Called Pethidine)

This narcotic is the most widely used pain-relief medication during childbirth throughout the world.[4] Demerol begins working to relieve your pain within five minutes if given via IV and within forty-five minutes if given by injection. The pain-relief effect typically lasts two and a half to three hours. Since the medication often causes nausea, it is usually given with an antinausea medication to fend off this side effect.

Ideally, Demerol should be used for pain relief more than four hours before birth. However, since labor is unpredictable, this is not always possible to plan. Babies born within two to three hours after the mother receives a dose of Demerol have been known to have an increased risk of respiratory depression (difficulty breathing).[5] The newborn may have the medication or breakdown products from the medication (called metabolites) in its blood for approximately a day and a half after birth.

Morphine

A drug that has been used for pain relief during childbirth for over a century, morphine lasts just as long as Demerol, and for all practical purposes is a very similar drug. Morphine is frequently used in IV pain relief, injections, and epidurals for cesarean delivery (although rarely used for epidurals during labor). The pain-relieving effects of morphine take place within three to five minutes after receiving the medication via an IV and within twenty to forty minutes if received by injection. Typically, the pain-relieving effect can last a few hours, depending on how labor is progressing and how well the laboring mom is coping. This medication may cause you to experience itching, constipation, nausea, drowsiness, and blurred vision.

Morphine crosses the placenta quickly, and there is a risk of respiratory depression in the newborns of mothers who have been given morphine during labor. The effect of morphine on the baby depends on the dose given to the laboring mother and the size and weight of the newborn.[6]

Fentanyl

This synthetic narcotic takes effect within five minutes when given through an IV, and its pain-relief benefits last for approximately forty-five minutes. This drug is almost never given via intramuscular injection. Some research has shown that women experience less nausea and vomiting with fentanyl than with Demerol, and Narcan (a drug sometimes used on babies to reverse the effect of the narcotic) was used less often in the babies of moms who were given fentanyl than in the babies of moms who used Demerol.[7]

Nubain (Also Known as Nalbuphine) and Stadol (Also Known as Butorphanol)

These narcotics are frequently used on the maternity unit as a pain-relief measure. They are similar to the other narcotics, but when these are given in high doses, they tend to produce fewer effects on breathing than do the other narcotics. When given via IV, Nubain and Stadol provide pain relief within two to three minutes and if given by injection the pain-relief benefit takes effect within fifteen minutes. The pain-relief effect of these narcotics can range from three to six hours in laboring women.

Nubain and Stadol have also been observed to cause less nausea and vomiting in women compared to Demerol, but they do tend to more frequently produce the side effects of dizziness and drowsiness.[8] Some women report feeling relaxed once they are given Nubain or Stadol but do not experience significant pain relief with these medications. Both of these drugs cross the placenta, and both can cause sleepy babies after birth.

THE POTENTIAL SIDE EFFECTS OF ANALGESICS

On You

You may experience any (or none) of the following side effects: light-headedness, nausea, slowed breathing, itching, or difficulty urinating while in labor, until the medications wear off. Narcotics given for pain relief may cause constipation for a couple of days after you give birth.

On Your Baby

The side effects your newborn may experience may vary. All healthy babies have the ability to metabolize the medications that have crossed the placenta into their bloodstream, but this ability is not as well developed in premature babies. It is not common for a baby to be adversely affected by the small amounts of medication that cross over from its mother during childbirth. However, some babies receive enough medication to slow down their breathing (respiratory functioning) and may need to be monitored closely or given Narcan, a medication that reverses the effect of the narcotic the mother received. Some of these babies may have a difficult time initiating breast-feeding.[9]

If Narcan is needed, it is given to the baby (not the mother) immediately after birth to block the effects of the narcotic. The chances of the baby experiencing respiratory depression depend on the size and timing of the dose given to the mother during labor. The larger the dose and the closer to birth, the greater the chances of respiratory depression in the newborn.

Neurobehavioral changes are also found in some babies whose mothers used analgesics during labor and birth. These neurobehavioral changes can typically include floppy muscle tone and difficulty with initial feeding.

Local Anesthetic Agents

Local anesthetic agents are pain-relief medications that are administered directly into the part of your body where the sensations need to be blocked in order to keep you comfortable. Local anesthetic agents are not systemic, meaning they do not affect your entire nervous system. The most common use of a local anesthetic is an injection into the outer part of the vaginal area (also known as the perineum) for the purpose of providing pain relief during an episiotomy; this injection of local anesthetic numbs only the outer vaginal area. (An epi-siotomy is a controversial procedure where a cut is made in the perineum, by the obstetrician, to prevent tearing and to allow for passage of the baby.) As described below, an alternative to the epidural, which also uses local anesthetic medications, is the pudendal block, used at the time of delivery. Another type of block, rarely used anymore, is the paracervical block, which in-volves an injection of local anesthetic into the tissues surround-ing the cervix.

MOST COMMONLY USED LOCAL ANESTHESIA DURING CHILDBIRTH

Lidocaine and Nesacaine are the two most commonly used drugs for regional anesthesia in a pudendal block.

THE PUDENDAL BLOCK

The pudendal block is an injection given into the vaginal wall, and it is most often used during birth when it appears for-ceps will be needed to assist in the birth of the baby. Although this sounds like a painful procedure, it typically does not cause much discomfort and the comfort it brings (numbness) to the vaginal and rectal area as the baby exits can be significant. The pudendal block does not relieve the pain of your contractions, since it does not affect the sensations in your uterus, but it does numb your vaginal and rectal area. The pudendal block can be used on its own, if you prefer no other medications during labor, but this type of block is only effective in the late stages of labor.

This type of local anesthetic can be used during the push-ing stage of labor to numb your perineal area and will not im-pair your ability to push. A pudendal block will not be given if the baby's head has descended too far down the birth canal.

What You May Feel with the Pudendal Block

You may or may not feel the needle injection. You will still feel your contractions, but the relief of pain in the vaginal and rectal area may make it less painful, or not painful at all, to push the baby out.

When Can You Get the Pudendal Block?

The pudendal block is given almost anytime during the second (pushing) stage of labor. It can take effect within one to thirty minutes after you receive the medication and can last from approximately thirty minutes to three or four hours, depending on the amount and concentration of the dose given.

THE POTENTIAL BENEFIT OF LOCAL ANESTHESIA DURING LABOR

• Pain relief without an injection into the spine.

POTENTIAL SIDE EFFECTS OF LOCAL ANESTHESIA

On You

Side effects associated with local anesthesia are uncommon. Much like the numbing injections routinely given by your dentist, these injections are rarely associated with any significant side effect.

On Your Baby

This pain-relief method has minimal or no effect on the baby, but on rare occasions, the baby's heart rate can slow down after a pudendal block.

Nitrous Oxide

Inhalation of the gas nitrous oxide is a popular method of pain control during labor in Britain, but it is not commonly used in the United States.

WHAT IT IS AND WHAT IT DOES

Nitrous oxide is a flavorless, odorless gas, typically mixed with oxygen, that is inhaled through a face mask or mouthpiece. It is not clear exactly how nitrous oxide works to reduce pain levels. Typically its use results in diminished pain, or a continued awareness of pain without feeling bothered by it.

Almost every hospital in Britain has nitrous oxide units built into its labor and delivery rooms. Nitrous oxide is commonly used in the United States in dental offices (laughing gas), but it has not yet gained popularity as a pain-relief option during labor in the United States.

HOW IT IS DONE AND HOW IT FEELS

Your nurse or anesthesiologist will instruct you on how to use the face mask or mouthpiece. The mask will not be attached to you while you inhale the gas. This is intentional and will prevent you from inhaling too much gas at once. If you become too drowsy as a result of the gas, you will no longer be able to hold the mask or mouthpiece to your face.

To benefit from the effects of nitrous oxide, you need to place the mask to your face and breathe deeply before your next contraction begins. It takes about thirty to sixty seconds for the gas to become most effective, so you should try to time your inhalations about thirty seconds before each contraction, or at the moment you begin to feel your next contraction.

The effect of nitrous oxide has been described as a kind of strange sensation of feeling the pain while at the same time feeling a sense of bliss. So, the pain may still exist for some women, but the gas may create a feeling of "Painful contraction? *Who cares?*"

WHEN CAN YOU RECEIVE NITROUS OXIDE?

If you are in one of the few U.S. hospitals where it is offered, you can receive it at any point in your labor.

Potential Benefits of Nitrous Oxide

- You have control over the frequency and dose you give yourself.
- There is rapid onset of pain relief (pain-relief effects of the gas take place within one minute or less).
- If you do not want an epidural or other pain-relief medications, nitrous oxide may help you manage your labor pain so you can achieve your goal.
- The gas may take enough of an edge off of your pain to keep you comfortable until you receive an epidural.
- Once you stop inhaling the gas, you no longer feel its effects.

Potential Limitations of Nitrous Oxide

- It may not provide effective pain relief.
- You may not like the light-headed or "spacey" sensation.
- Some women do not like having to self-administer the gas and do not like the sensation of the mask on their face.
- The gas can make you feel dizzy or drowsy.
- If used for a long period over the course of labor, it can make you feel fatigued.
- Once you stop inhaling the gas, you no longer feel its effects.

Potential Side Effects of Nitrous Oxide

On You

- The gas can cause nausea and vomiting.
- Very rarely, if too much gas is inhaled, it can result in a loss of consciousness.

On Your Baby

- No adverse clinical side effects are known to impact the newborn.

A Caregiver's Perspective

We asked for perspectives from both an American and British anesthesiologist. Since, as we mentioned, nitrous oxide is widely used in England, we thought you might like to hear two points of view.

Mark Rosen, M.D., an anesthesiologist at the University of California, San Francisco

"Nitrous oxide has played an important role and has been extremely helpful in my practice over the past two decades. I believe, much like narcotics, the pain may seem the same, but the patient doesn't care as much about it. You might think of nitrous oxide as a patient-controlled inhalation analgesia. One reason for its success is the element of control it gives to women during labor.

"Sometimes, it seems as though the use of nitrous oxide is merely an appetizer before the epidural. Although I have never considered it to be an agent/technique to replace epidural analgesia, I have found its use wonderful for some women, particularly toward the end of the first stage of labor or in the second (pushing) stage of labor."

Felicity Plaat, M.D., an anesthesiologist at Queen Charlotte's Hospital, London, describing her use of nitrous oxide on the maternity unit

"I am quite a fan of the use of nitrous oxide for pain relief during labor. I think it is particularly useful for repeat moms and for first-time moms who are waiting for an epidural. As well as providing pain relief, some women really enjoy the 'laughing gas' effect. In fact, I came across one couple where she puffed away during each contraction, only to hand the tubing over to her partner between contractions. There's togetherness!

"The disadvantage of this method: some women find it is tiring if used over a long period, and you need to get the timing right for its full effect."

What Women Say About Pain-Relief Medications During Childbirth

Shelley Fisher, a mother of two, who used a narcotic for the birth of her second child

Why Did You Decide to Use Nubain?
"I decided to use Nubain because I had been given this drug with my first child and had liked it. Who knows, it was probably the narcotic effect, but it relaxed me enough so that I could start to enjoy the process and anticipate the delivery. Before being given Nubain, I could feel my anxiety and fear with each contraction."

Did It Provide Pain Relief?
"I asked for Nubain once I was four to five centimeters dilated, immediately after I heard my husband order meatloaf for me from the hospital dietician, who had the unfortunate timing of stepping into the room just as I was wracked with the first long and extremely intense contraction of my labor. After I recovered from the contraction, I chastised my husband for his choice of dinner (Meatloaf? I was giving birth on Easter Sunday!). He strongly suggested I order something for the pain! The Nubain did relieve the painful contractions for about one hour."

Partner Involvement
"My husband was very supportive of my using anything to control and relieve the pain."

*Did You Use Any Other Comfort Measures or
Pain-Relief Interventions?*

"I tried to use a birth ball at one point. Fortunately, a nurse
came in to tell me that I was using it wrong and showed me
how to use it. I was having some back labor at that point, which
the birth ball helped, but it did not dull the contractions."

*Do You Think the Relief of Your Pain Impacted
Your Satisfaction with Your Birth?*

"I did not have an epidural during this birth, as I did for the
delivery of my first child, because I was told there wasn't
enough time. Given the personality of my younger child, it
shouldn't have surprised me, looking back, that he had such an
explosive delivery. I feel strongly that if I had experienced less
pain during his birth, the whole experience would have been
much better. When I learned that I would not be getting an
epidural, my anxiety rose tenfold; I was terrified of the pain.
That fear dampened and clouded my anticipation for the birth
of my baby. My memory of this delivery is not one of easy
labor and bliss, but one of explosive pain and fear."

**Marsha Song, a mother of three who used a narcotic
during the birth of her first baby**

Why Did You Decide to Use Pain Medications?

"I did not specifically request Stadol for my pain, but it was
suggested as a method to control pain during labor. This was
my first delivery and I was willing to try it because I had hopes
for giving birth without an epidural."

Was It What You Expected?

"No. I was having severe back labor and I was told that it
would 'take the edge off.' In fact, it made me extremely sleepy.
I found myself dozing between contractions only to be awakened by the extreme pain of the next contraction. The Stadol
seemed to intensify the pain because the dozing prevented me

from preparing for the next contraction. It made me so tired, I wasn't sure I could get through the labor. It was a horrible experience for me."

Did You Use Any Other Comfort Measures or Pain-Relief Interventions?

"I had an epidural after the Stadol experience. I was having such difficult back labor. I had no complications with the epidural except that I was completely numb from the chest down [this was in 1996] and at first I could not feel to help push. My obstetrician wanted to use forceps but I was against it. I was finally able to push the baby out without assistance."

Donna Shore, a mother of one child, describing her experience with narcotic pain relief during the birth of her baby

Why Did You Decide to Use Nubain?

"I tried to soothe my labor pain with a warm whirlpool bath. It wasn't long before I realized that the pain was too strong and I would not be able to go forward without some relief. I asked for an epidural but was told it was too late for one, but that I could receive Nubain."

Did It Provide Pain Relief?

"Nubain did help me relax, but once my contractions became really strong I do not know how much it helped. The bottom line is that it did not provide enough pain relief."

Did You Use Any Other Comfort Measures or Pain-Relief Interventions?

"I tried to use music and the whirlpool bath as instructed by the Bradley method, but these things did nothing to comfort me. I would not use Nubain again as my first line of defense for pain, since it was not effective enough for the pain of my contractions."

*Do You Think the Relief of Your Pain Impacted
Your Satisfaction with Your Birth?*

"Definitely. I was so focused on going through the contraction that I could not concentrate on anything else and consequently I do not remember much about the delivery. After this experience, I pledged that if I ever had another baby I would use whatever medications were available, as soon as possible."

Six

COMPLEMENTARY AND ALTERNATIVE APPROACHES TO LABOR-PAIN RELIEF

Which Ones Relieve Your Pain and Which Ones Just Help You Cope (and When It Makes a Difference)

Alternatives to traditional medical interventions, such as water immersion and the use of hypnosis and aromatherapy, to name just a few, are becoming increasingly common, particularly in women's health care and during childbirth. When these alternative techniques are used in addition to traditional medical pain-relief methods, it is called *complementary medicine*. When these techniques are used instead of the traditional medical approach, it is known as *alternative medicine*. Increasingly, many women are seeking a variety of ways to address the pain of childbirth by integrating both complementary and alternative methods. This combination of complementary and alternative medicine is referred to as *CAM*.

CAM is defined as "medical interventions not taught widely at U.S. medical schools nor generally available at U.S. hospitals," according to the National Center for Complementary and Alternative Medicine of the National Institutes of

Health. However, many of the CAM approaches for pain management during childbirth are increasingly becoming available on hospital labor and delivery units throughout the country.

All of the methods described in this chapter can be used on their own, without any form of medical pain relief, or they can be used to complement the various forms of medical pain relief available during childbirth. The breathing and relaxation techniques that have been a cornerstone of hospital childbirth preparation courses since the 1970s are examples of complementary (and sometimes alternative) forms of pain management.

It is to your advantage to understand many of these nonmedical approaches to childbirth, even if you feel you will want to use an epidural or other pain-relief medications. Circumstances can arise that may prevent or delay the use of pain-relief medications—for instance, if your labor progresses more quickly than you had anticipated—and your knowledge of nonmedical pain-management methods may provide you with comfort in these situations.

How Are CAMs Used During Childbirth?

Some women find that one (or more) of these nonmedical pain-relief measures can provide an effective way to cope with the pain of early labor, until they are ready to receive medical pain relief. Some find that a particular CAM method may actually diminish their pain level during labor or birth, making it possible for them to delay or even avoid the use of pain-relief medications, if that is their goal. And others may choose to use nonmedical pain-relief methods exclusively during childbirth, whether or not these methods prove effective in reducing their pain level.

Some of these methods may reduce labor pain in some women, but in general, most of these CAM approaches do not significantly reduce or eliminate the pain of labor in childbirth, and most do not claim to. Many of the proponents and educators of these CAM childbirth methods do not suggest that your childbirth experience will be pain-free. Instead, the emphasis is on teaching you a technique or skill that is meant to provide you with the tools needed to deal with the pain of childbirth.

The degree of effectiveness associated with each of the CAM approaches to pain management can vary depending upon a variety of factors, such as your own pain threshold, the intensity of your individual labor pain, the amount of preparation or practice you've had, and the type and strength of support available to you during labor.

WHEN DOES IT MAKE A DIFFERENCE?

Your birth philosophy, or your beliefs and values regarding the experience of childbirth, determines how you view your labor pain. Some of the CAMs used to manage labor pain are less pain-relief "technique" than they are birth "philosophy." For instance, women who believe that the experience of coping with labor pain holds value, physically, emotionally, and spiritually, may be committed to using absolutely no pain medications, even if the complementary or alternative methods do not significantly reduce their pain level. They may find reward and satisfaction in continuing to deal with labor pain, as long as they are able to achieve their goal of an unmedicated birth. On the other hand, women who wish to reduce or eliminate pain during childbirth may discontinue the use of a nonmedical approach that does not provide adequate pain relief.

Generally speaking, women may experience three common outcomes when they choose to use CAM approaches during labor and birth.

1. Women who have a strong preference to experience childbirth with as little pain as possible may use one or more CAM techniques successfully during early labor. Once labor intensifies, and pain grows more severe, they

may find the CAM approach inadequate to keep them comfortable, and opt for medical pain relief to achieve the type of birth experience they desire.

2. Some women want to use only CAM methods but find that their pain is more intense than they had anticipated. At some point in their labor, they change their minds and opt to use a medical pain-relief method.

3. Some women are prepared and committed to using CAM techniques consistent with their birth philosophy. Regardless of the pain factor, they are able to achieve a rewarding, satisfying labor and birth.

This chapter is divided into two sections. The first section describes the approaches using CAMs that are typically regarded as birth philosophies (rather than specific pain-management techniques).

CAM Birth Philosophies

- The Lamaze philosophy and the Bradley method— both have influenced childbirth education courses for decades.
- Water immersion and waterbirth. Is this really the "Wet epidural"?
- Hypnosis—your mind's power to overcome your body's experience of pain and discomfort.

The second section describes CAMs that are usually regarded as methods used to provide comfort, support, and pain management to laboring women.

CAM Pain-Management Methods

- Acupuncture—a centuries-old and fascinating approach to pain management.
- Labor support—a little TLC goes a long way.
- Aromatherapy—the therapeutic use of scent.
- Sterile water papules—specifically for back labor.

- Transcutaneous electrical nerve stimulation (TENS)—the "electrical massage."
- The birth ball—used for movement and repositioning.

LAMAZE®

What It Is and What It Does

Lamaze childbirth preparation has been around since the 1960s, but it did not become a mainstay in American hospitals until the 1970s. Dr. Fernand Lamaze, a French physician, named this method of childbirth "childbirth without pain." This technique, formerly called psychoprophylaxis, uses various strategies (typically breathing and relaxation techniques) to prevent pain. Lamaze educators today do not claim that Lamaze is a pain-free birth approach. Today's Lamaze birth philosophy promotes the belief that birth is normal, natural, and healthy—that there is value to your labor pain since it prompts you to become active in ways that may enhance the birth process, through movement, breathing, and using focused concentration. Lamaze is still a cornerstone of most hospital-based childbirth education courses today, and classes are taught by Lamaze-certified childbirth educators in a variety of other settings as well. Lamaze-certified childbirth educators are certified by Lamaze International, the only childbirth educator program accredited by the National Organization for Competency Assurance (NOCA).

In addition to breathing and concentration, Lamaze classes also cover the use of other coping strategies, which can include labor support, massage, and hydrotherapy. Lamaze classes also benefit women who may opt for medical pain relief. According to Linda Harmon, the executive director of Lamaze International, "The Lamaze approach to birth recognizes that women's inner wisdom will guide them to confidently respond to labor and to use strategies to increase their comfort level during childbirth."

Lamaze is by far the most recognizable childbirth approach in this country. Although Lamaze is often thought of as a specific breathing technique used during labor, Lamaze childbirth preparation has evolved over the last decade from teaching a method for giving birth to promoting an entire philosophy that provides "a foundation and direction for women as they prepare to give birth and become mothers."[1]

The Lamaze International Position Paper, *Lamaze for the 21st Century,* states: "Ultimately, the goal of Lamaze classes is that every woman gives birth confidently, free to find comfort in a wide variety of ways, and supported by family and health care professionals who trust that she has within her the ability to give birth."[2] The Lamaze philosophy maintains that the following care practices promote, support, and protect nature's plan for birth:

1. Labor begins on its own.
2. Freedom of movement throughout labor.
3. Continuous labor support.
4. No routine interventions (procedures that are done due to hospital protocol or policy, and not in response to a specific medical concern).
5. Nonsupine (upright or side-lying) positions for birth.
6. No separation of mother and baby after birth with unlimited opportunity for breast-feeding.[3]

How It Works and How It Feels
The Lamaze philosophy emphasizes that birth requires active participation and promotes the use of various strategies to remain comfortable as labor intensifies. It recognizes that most women require more than simple breathing and focusing techniques to respond to the intensity of labor. Lamaze certified childbirth educators encourage women to work actively with

labor, finding comfort in response to their body's discomfort or pain through the use of any or all of the following activities:

- walking
- rocking and position changes
- massage
- hydrotherapy
- the use of birth balls
- focal point concentration (focusing on an object or image)
- an active birth partner or spouse who participates with you in the implementation of the above techniques and provides comfort and support.[4]

Each of these strategies may provide comfort for some women, while others may find them less effective.

Why Women Choose Lamaze
Women who choose to give birth using the Lamaze philosophy have the primary objective of giving birth with as few medical interventions as possible, and of having a childbirth experience in which they feel equipped to effectively manage and cope with their labor pain.

Most women learn about Lamaze through friends, family, health care providers, or in their childbirth preparation courses. Women choosing to attend Lamaze classes will find they are based on the following tenets of the Lamaze philosophy of birth:

- Birth is normal, natural, and healthy.
- The experience of birth profoundly affects women and their families.
- Women's inner wisdom guides them through birth.
- Women's confidence and ability to give birth is either enhanced or diminished by the care provider and place of birth.
- Women have the right to give birth free from routine medical interventions.

- Birth can safely take place in birth centers and homes.
- Childbirth education empowers women to make informed choices in health care, to assume responsibility for their health, and to trust their inner wisdom.[5]

Your Partner's Role

Your partner will play an important role in labor support with the strategies learned in Lamaze classes. He will be taught how to support you through your labor, as you use the coping methods listed earlier.

Potential Benefits of Lamaze

- The strategies used to remain active during labor may promote relaxation and, in some women, may lessen the pain of labor.
- Labor support is a vital part of the process, and your partner or a doula can help you use these techniques during labor.
- You will learn about natural pain-management options as well as medical pain-relief options.
- Lamaze can be used in conjunction with almost every other pain-management method.

Potential Limitations of Lamaze

- These strategies and techniques may not provide adequate pain relief.
- You must be committed to gaining the knowledge, skills, and support to benefit from the strategies offered.

RESEARCH SAYS: *In one survey in which over sixty Lamaze-prepared moms were interviewed, the majority of women in the survey (95 percent) reported that being informed about labor and delivery (through the Lamaze approach) was valuable because it decreased their fear and increased their relaxation, reduced their tension, and increased their chances of managing their labor well.*[6]

A Caregiver's Perspective

Biddy Fein, a certified nurse-midwife, and a Lamaze-certified childbirth educator, who served on the Lamaze International board of directors for six years

"Childbirth is normal and women have the ability to birth within them. In the media, childbirth is fraught with crisis and hysteria, which is anything but normal. Women in our culture are not taught to be confident and do not necessarily believe that birth is a normal process. By learning from childbirth educators who subscribe to the Lamaze philosophy, families are empowered to birth with confidence and to be active participants in their own care. The role of the childbirth educator as advocate is an important one that helps women become good consumers of health care for themselves and ultimately for their families."

What Women Say About Lamaze

Georgie Marks Magner, a Lamaze mom, a Lamaze instructor, and the state coordinator for Lamaze International, Massachusetts

Why Did You Decide to Use Lamaze?

"I actively sought out a Lamaze class for my second child after a disappointing and unsatisfying birth experience with my first child. I went into this birth confident that I had prepared enough to know how to handle the contractions and pain of labor and how I wanted to deliver my baby."

How Was Your Partner Involved?

"I had an active support person (my husband) with me the entire time. It was a very intense labor, and a quick labor, like my first, but I was able to relax, and I moved around, sitting, squatting, kneeling throughout the labor while my husband assisted me with lots of massage, breathing assistance, and humor."

Were You Satisfied with Your Lamaze Birth?

"After the birth, my son was so alert, he nursed well, and I felt as if I was on top of the world. I was out of bed walking around, taking a shower and having breakfast within an hour of giving birth. My body was sore and tired (it felt somewhat like it did when I swam the 1,650-yard master's swimming competition) but emotionally I felt great. It was wonderful. I still get a warm fuzzy feeling every time I think of that birth experience."

Cheryl Donahue, a Lamaze instructor and mother of ten children

Why Did You Decide to Use Lamaze?

"I have experienced seven unmedicated births and three Pitocin-induced epidural births. I prefer the unmedicated births hands down. The reasons I was able to give birth without medication are simple: I had terrific support, felt safe, was able to relax and breathe, and let my body go with the contractions."

How Was Your Partner Involved?

"The epitome of all of these criteria was evident in the labor and birth of my fifth child. During most of the labor it-self, my doctor, a very dear friend, my husband, and the nurse were in the room. Because of their presence I felt safe and supported even within a large city hospital."

Did the Methods Used in the Lamaze Birth Philosophy Provide Pain Relief?

"I was able to completely relax my body and visualize my uterus pushing my baby out. The slow, relaxed Lamaze breathing saw me through much of this."

Were You Satisfied with Your Lamaze Birth?

"The birth itself, as with all my unmedicated births, was absolutely, ecstatically joyful, and yes, empowering. I was able to push a fifteen-and-a-half-inch head out of my body and then get up and walk around afterward. Breast-feeding and gazing into an unmedicated newborn's eyes is in itself a miracle!"

Resources

Lamaze International
2025 M Street, NW, Suite 800
Washington, D.C. 20036
www.lamaze.org

THE BRADLEY METHOD—HUSBAND-COACHED CHILDBIRTH

What It Is and What It Does

Today, it is assumed that your husband or partner will play an important role during your childbirth experience, but until the 1960s, in most hospitals, husbands were not permitted in the labor and delivery room. Dr. Robert A. Bradley, an obstetrician and natural childbirth proponent, believed women should have a natural, drug-free childbirth experience in which their husbands played an active role. Dr. Bradley's inclusion of the husband in the childbirth experience was regarded as quite radical and met with plenty of resistance.

The Bradley method teaches the husband or partner how to coach the mother with her breathing, to help her to achieve and maintain a state of relaxation, and to assist in keeping the birth environment free of distractions. It stresses the importance of good nutrition for pregnant women, recommends specific exercises during pregnancy, and teaches Dr. Bradley's deep-breathing methods, which he termed sleep-breathing, to be used for pain management throughout labor. The Bradley method promotes the belief that if women have knowledge and understanding about why childbirth causes pain, they will be less fearful during labor and better able to cope with their pain.

The Bradley method is taught by certified instructors in a course that is typically twelve weeks long. The classes are usually very small and intimate, with no more than eight couples to a class. The relaxation techniques taught in class were developed to help women cope with labor pain, and the release of tension through the deep-breathing techniques may help reduce the experience of labor pain for some women. The Bradley method does not claim to offer a pain-free birth experience, but provides women with the techniques needed to manage their pain level to reach their goal of achieving an unmedicated birth experience.

> It is estimated that over a half million couples have used the Bradley method.[7]

Why You Would Choose the Bradley Method

- You are committed to avoiding the use of pain-relief medications throughout your childbirth experience.
- The Bradley instructors have an especially high rate of moms who successfully use this method without requesting an epidural or other pain-relief medications. To some women, this success rate may make the Bradley method more appealing than other pain-management methods.
- You would like your partner to actively participate in the birth experience with you.

Potential Benefits

- The Bradley method can be used effectively in any birth setting: home, birth center, or hospital.
- There are no known risks associated with this method.
- Your husband or partner actively participates with you throughout the birth process.
- The Bradley techniques are easy to learn.
- The Bradley method covers all of the material taught in most childbirth preparation courses, so you do not have to attend additional courses.

Potential Limitations

- If pain management becomes an issue during your labor, you may find that you need to use additional pain-relief methods.
- You will need to commit to twelve "units" of instruction to learn the Bradley method over a period of twelve continuous weeks.
- Since the Bradley method rejects the use of pain-relief medications, women who embrace this method but end up requesting an epidural or other pain-relief medications during labor may feel disappointed in their birth experience.

A Caregiver's Perspective

Laura Conrad, a certified Bradley instructor who has used the Bradley Method during the births of her two children

"Labor is the only time in our lives when the experience of intense pain does not signify a problem within our bodies; we are accustomed to reacting to pain with fear. The Bradley method provides women with the knowledge and understanding of why our bodies feel pain during childbirth. This knowledge and understanding help reduce our fear, leaving us better able to deal with the work of labor.

"The Bradley method sets realistic expectations for women. We tell you there is going to be intense pain, but we tell you *why* this is so and teach you and your partner various techniques that allow you both to participate in successfully managing your labor pain. The Bradley method teaches the husband or partner how to provide emotional support to the laboring mother by providing encouragement and praise, and if women begin to feel overwhelmed by their contractions, they remind them of why they chose not to give birth using medical pain-relief methods, and help them to try to maintain focus and determination to stay with the Bradley method.

"Any woman can decide to use the Bradley method, but there are commonalities among women who find this birth approach more desirable than others. Many women choose the Bradley method because they are independent by nature and do not want their birth experience managed by others. Lots of Bradley moms have a strong sense of empowerment and are determined to give birth using their inner strength and resources. Others who come to the Bradley method are very physically active and prefer a natural approach to almost all aspects of their lives, including their birth experience. Some seek out the Bradley method for religious reasons; giving birth naturally is consistent with their religious beliefs."

What Women Say About the Bradley Method

Ellen Kuppinger, whose first baby was born using the Bradley Method

Why Did You Decide to Use the Bradley Method?
"It was very important to me to experience childbirth as women have before me for hundreds of thousands of years. I wanted to feel the pain that childbirth brings; I wanted to feel the muscles of my uterus working to push my baby out into the world. I felt that numbing my body to the pain would be cheating myself out of a very special experience."

Did the Bradley Method Provide Pain Relief?

"I was not looking for pain relief. The Bradley method helped me manage the pain; the breathing relaxed my body and helped me deal with it better. For a few contractions I tensed up at the height of them, and that made it far worse than relaxing and riding the contractions."

Would You Use the Bradley Method Again?

"I absolutely would use the Bradley method again, and I recommend it to every woman. I encourage every woman to experience childbirth *with* pain. It is amazing to feel what your body is capable of."

Kimberly G. Bell, the mother of three babies born using the Bradley Method

Was Your Labor What You Expected?

"The labor experience is never exactly what you envision. You have to prepare and educate yourself so you are ready for any and all scenarios. It is painful, trying at times, and emotionally jam-packed, but the hopeful result is the same for every mom and couple—a healthy baby and healthy mom.

"Not only were my children born completely drug-free without intervention, but I achieved my greatest feelings of accomplishment by laboring and then delivering my children naturally. I would not trade anything for those experiences, or sacrifice the benefits for my children, gained by a natural pregnancy and birth."

Did the Bradley Method Provide Pain Relief?

"You focus on the pain, knowing that it is bringing you closer to seeing your baby and that you are doing it all to give your baby the best start you can. Pain is something you need to focus on whether it is a little or a lot. All through labor you need to manage your pain through the encouragement from your Bradley partner; relaxation techniques; a shower, bath or

whirlpool; music; massage of pressure points; various laboring positions; and unyielding support during each and every
contraction."

*Would You Use the Bradley Method Again? Would
You Recommend This Method to Other Women?*
"Yes. Absolutely. I would wholeheartedly recommend the
Bradley method to everyone. Even if you are not able to have a
natural birth (or don't want to), the benefit of the classes in
terms of educating yourself about labor and delivery is so
tremendous that I simply don't understand why every woman
in America has not taken them or planned to. Natural childbirth is an amazing, delicate, and miraculous event that should
not simply be brushed aside because of a misconception that it
is simply 'too painful.' "

**Jennifer Downie, who used the Bradley Method for the
birth of her first baby**

Why Did You Decide to Use the Bradley Method?
"I have significant experience in the practice of yoga. The
breathing methods and general philosophy of the Bradley
method are consistent with my previous yoga training."

Was It What You Expected?
"The Bradley classes were much more helpful than I could
have ever expected, but labor, delivery, and recovery were
worse than I expected. I began to have back labor three days
prior to my actual delivery. I used the positions and relaxation
methods suggested in my class to try to be more comfortable. I
did experience some relief with these techniques, but by the
third day I was getting very tired."

Did the Bradley Method Provide Pain Relief?
"Although I do feel that avoiding pain medication is a
worthwhile objective, there is so much more to the Bradley
method than just avoiding pain medication. If my highest ob-

jective was to experience delivery without the use of pain relief, I was not successful. However, the Bradley classes provided a great deal of other information that allowed me to feel very satisfied with my experience, in spite of the fact that, before I became completely exhausted, I accepted the use of Pitocin and pain medication (a narcotic and an epidural) to help me deliver the baby."

Heather Vaz, who used the Bradley Method for the birth of her first baby

Was Your Labor What You Expected?

"The Bradley classes prepared me very well about pregnancy, labor, and childbirth. The knowledge I gained was instrumental in having the childbirth we wanted."

Did the Bradley Method Provide Pain Relief?

"The Bradley method did not provide pain relief, but it did provide my husband and me with the tools to make it through labor and childbirth. I definitely felt every pain and had severe back labor, which I was not expecting. I used the relaxation techniques that we had learned (and my husband and I had practiced) to get me through each contraction. I used a whirlpool tub as well and labored mostly at home because it is a more comfortable environment. (I was at the hospital one and a half hours before my son arrived.)

"I also managed pain with whatever felt best—which for me was moaning. My doctor said I was speaking in tongues, but it helped me get through each contraction. In addition to the warm Jacuzzi bath, I also used the birth ball, a massage tool, and watched a funny movie while laboring at home."

Resources

American Academy of Husband-Coached Childbirth
P.O. Box 5224

Sherman Oaks, CA 91413-5224
www.bradleybirth.com

LABORING IN WATER AND WATERBIRTH

What It Is and What It Does

Hydrotherapy is the use of water to relieve pain during labor, and can specifically refer to anything from standing under a warm shower to the use of tubs and whirlpools to immersing yourself in a birthing pool to bring comfort during labor.

Many maternity units are beginning to encourage women to spend time in the shower or tub for relaxation and comfort during labor. More hospitals are installing private showers in their birthing rooms. The use of a birthing pool during labor is a more recent development and is gaining in popularity in the United States: many hospitals and birth centers are now installing birthing pools to provide laboring women with another option for pain management. Today most women who labor in the birthing pool leave the pool when they are ready to deliver the baby.

> **DID YOU KNOW?** *"In 1995 two U.S. hospitals offered waterbirths; today over 120 hospitals have had at least one water birth and more hospitals are offering the use of showers for relief and comfort during labor."*[8]

Waterbirth, or actually giving birth in water, is a fairly new approach to childbirth and is not as common in the United States as it is in some European countries, but it is on the rise here, with more hospitals providing trained staff and birthing pools than ever before. Not all hospitals that provide birthing pools for laboring women allow women to give birth in the pool. If you would like the option of giving birth in water, you should check with your hospital to make sure it is able to accommodate your preference.

> A birthing pool or tub should be filled with at least eighteen inches of water for the laboring woman to achieve the buoyancy needed for effective pain relief.

How It Is Done and How It Feels

Hospitals and birth centers that provide the use of a birthing pool will have their own guidelines (protocols) that determine how the mother should labor and/or give birth in the pool. The birthing pool itself is a large whirlpool-type tub, usually deep enough for you to fully immerse yourself sitting down. Some pools have water jets; others do not. The temperature is usually kept between 95 and 101 degrees Fahrenheit and is checked regularly by the nurse or midwife to ensure that it does not exceed or drop below this temperature, as a safety precaution to you and your newborn.

Only women who are at least thirty-seven weeks pregnant and regarded as low risk (meaning there are no complications or health issues known to exist in either you or your baby) are currently allowed to labor and, in some hospitals and birth centers, give birth in water. You will be screened by your nurse, physician, or midwife to determine whether there is any reason that you should not labor or give birth in water. If it's a go, you will enter the pool with the assistance of a nurse or midwife, who will stay with you while you soak.

The timing of when women are encouraged to enter and leave the pool can vary among hospitals and birth centers. Some may require you to reach a specific point of dilation (or to be in active labor) before entering the pool, to avoid the risk of slowing down your labor. Other hospitals and birth centers are more flexible on this issue and encourage women to enter the pool for pain relief whenever they feel ready. You may leave the pool at any time during labor, and you will never be left alone while you are in the pool. In hospitals that do not allow for the baby to be born underwater, you will need to get out of the pool to deliver the baby. (Don't worry, your nurse, midwife, or physician will help you with the timing on that one.) Every hospital or birth center that offers waterbirth as an option should have midwives and/or physicians specifically trained and experienced in waterbirths.

You and your baby will be monitored as needed, or according to your hospital's protocol, in the birthing pool. Your baby's heartbeat can be monitored with a waterproof device (a Doppler) that your caregiver can apply to your belly while you are in the tub. Usually during active labor, your nurse or midwife will listen to the baby's heartbeat every thirty minutes, for one minute. If additional monitoring is needed at any point in your labor, you will be asked to get out of the pool but may return if your caregiver determines that all is well with you and your baby.

DID YOU KNOW? *Women who use water immersion during the first stage of labor report significantly less pain than women who do not labor in water.*[9]

Many women who have used water immersion during labor have found that the soothing and calming effect of the water allowed them to feel more relaxed, even when their pain persisted. For these women, although their pain continued, their state of relaxation and the peaceful feelings experienced as a result of water immersion helped them stay focused on coping with their labor pain.

DID YOU KNOW? *One survey of women who opted for waterbirth showed that women who chose to labor and birth in water desired a drug-free method of reducing pain and a gentle birth experience for their newborn. Many felt more in control of their birth environment and especially appreciated the relaxing, calming effect of the water.*[10]

Your Partner's Role During Water Immersion or Waterbirth

Your partner can play an active role by providing you with massage and simply by being present while you labor. Some hospitals and birth centers allow the partner to enter the pool with the laboring mother.

Potential Benefits of Water Immersion or Waterbirth

- Some women report relief from labor pain once they enter the water.
- Some women report that their labor pain is not diminished, but the calming, soothing effect of the water helps them cope with the pain.
- Many women report an enhanced ability to concentrate and focus once they enter the water.
- Since you are more buoyant in water, water immersion allows for easy repositioning and movement.
- Water immersion can be combined with other comfort methods, such as massage and aromatherapy.

Potential Limitations of Water Immersion or Waterbirth

The most commonly cited limitations to using water immersion are:

- You are unable to use narcotics or an epidural for additional pain relief while laboring in the pool.

- You can't wear that pretty hospital johnny while in the pool. (Some women wear just a comfortable T-shirt or sports bra; others prefer to wear nothing at all.)

Conditions or Situations That May Prevent You from Using Water Immersion or Having a Waterbirth (Depending on the Guidelines Used by Your Hospital or Birth Center)

- You are having twins.
- Your baby is in the breech position (bottom first rather than head first).
- Your baby is premature or there is the threat of premature labor.
- The second stage of labor—the pushing stage—becomes very long, as determined by your midwife or obstetrician.
- You have previously had a cesarean section.
- Your labor has been induced (you received oxytocin).
- You have received a narcotic within the last six hours.
- You have active genital herpes.
- You have an infection such as HIV, hepatitis B or C,★ or you have tested positive for Group B streptococcus.
- You have a fever or there is a question of possible infection.
- You have meconium-stained amniotic fluid (you may be allowed to labor, but not deliver, in the pool).
- Your bag of waters has broken (ruptured membranes).†
- You have excessive vaginal bleeding.
- You have any condition that requires continuous electronic fetal heart rate monitoring.

★ There is a difference of opinion among caregivers regarding the threat of infection to the newborn (or to others using the bath) when the laboring woman is known to have an infection. Many hospitals prevent women with any kind of infection, including HIV, hepatitis B or C, and Group B streptococcus from using the pool or bath during labor.
† Some hospitals prohibit women from laboring in the pool or bath when their bag of waters has broken (ruptured membranes). However, there is currently no evidence of increased infection with or without ruptured membranes.

You will be asked to leave the pool if:

• Your baby is showing distress.
• You desire medical pain relief such as a narcotic or an epidural.
• Your labor is progressing very slowly.
• You start bleeding during labor.
• You begin to feel faint.
• Your temperature exceeds 100.4 degrees Fahrenheit.

IMMERSION IN WATER DURING LABOR AND BIRTH: CONCERNS AND CONTROVERSY

Potential Risks

The two most common concerns raised by some caregivers regarding waterbirth are the risk of the newborn drowning or breathing in water during birth and the increased risk of infection to both mother and newborn. Although it has been suggested that more studies need to be conducted, there is currently no evidence that babies born in water have a higher mortality rate than babies born on dry land, and the rate of infection in babies born in water is the same as in babies born on land.

The Risk of Baby Breathing in Water

It is thought that a variety of physical processes prevents the newborn from attempting to breathe underwater; until the baby reaches the surface, it is not stimulated to breathe. At birth the baby's head is immediately raised to the surface of the water, where, upon sensing the change in the environment from water to air, the baby takes its first breath.

> **RESEARCH SAYS:** *Two large studies conducted in England found similar results. The more recent study, conducted between 1994 and 1996, which traced the outcomes of over four thousand waterbirths, determined that the percentage of babies who were admitted to the special care unit for complications after birth was the same as for babies born to low-risk mothers who did not have a waterbirth. The study also found that the mortality rates for babies born in water were not higher than the mortality rates of those born on land.*[11]
>
> *The other study, conducted between 1989 and 1994, determined that there were no significant differences in the number of babies who had to be admitted to the special care unit among the babies born in water and the babies born on dry land.*[12]

The Risk of Infection

Presently, there is no research indicating that the risk of infection is higher for either the mother or baby by laboring or giving birth in water. Some caregivers and birthing mothers have concerns that the babies might be exposed to a greater risk of infection by being born into water, or some may worry about this even if the moms only labor—but do not give birth—in water. After each use, the birthing pool is thoroughly cleaned and disinfected with a solution that guards against the risk of spreading infection.

One study on this issue concluded: "Waterbirth nowadays is one of the legitimate methods of alternative obstetrics. The results of our study did confirm that this way of delivery does not represent any risk for the mother or the newborn and that there is no reason for anxiety of obstetrician and neonatologist."[13]

Another study that evaluated waterbirths and other forms of alternative birthing concluded that these births "do not demonstrate higher birth risks for the mother or the child than bedbirths if the same medical criteria are used in the monitoring as well as in the management of birth."[14]

Does Water Immersion or Waterbirth Provide Effective Pain Relief?

Some studies suggest that women who labor and give birth in water are less likely to request medical pain relief. Other studies have suggested that the use of pain-relief medications did not differ among women who labored in water and those who did not. While it may be true that many women who choose water immersion or waterbirth do not use as many medications as those who do not labor in water, it is important to note that most women who choose to labor in water already place a high value on a drug-free birth experience. Thus, for some women, the reduction in drug use with this type of birth may not necessarily be as a result of the pain relief provided by the water immersion.

One important recent study on the use of water immersion evaluated the rates of epidural usage and cesarean deliveries among women in the first stage of labor who were diagnosed with dystocia (when cervical dilation stops or slows down to less than one centimeter per hour). The findings of this study suggest that immersion in water during labor resulted in fewer requests for epidural pain relief, no increase in the length of labor compared to women who did not use water immersion, and no increase in the need for the use of forceps to assist in the birth of the baby. In addition, women in the study who used water immersion, compared to those who did not, reported less pain and increased satisfaction. There was no difference in rate of cesarean delivery between the two groups.[15]

In a separate review, however, which compared the birth experience of close to one thousand women who used water immersion with women who did not, there were no statistically different outcomes shown for use of pain relief, length of first stage of labor, or perineal injury (vaginal tearing). There were no significant differences in Apgar scores and infection rates of newborns.[16]

The women in our interviews who have described their use of water immersion during labor report a variety of responses.

Some found immersion in water reduced the intensity of their labor pain; others found it did not, but the comfort of the water allowed them to effectively manage their pain.

According to most of the current research done on this method, low-risk pregnant women who labor or birth in water, under the supervision of an experienced caregiver, fare just as well as, and sometimes better than, women who choose not to use water during labor or birth.

A Caregiver's Perspective

Brooke Arnold, a certified professional midwife and doula in Dallas, Texas, who frequently uses water immersion in her practice

"Water is a must-have for your bag of pain-relief tricks. With the right timing, water can even provide enough pain relief to eliminate your need for medication. I offer water to women in active labor when their own coping techniques are no longer working, and it usually takes them right through transition. The pain relief from water is immediate and allows them to re-focus and cope with contractions again. When I take laboring women out of the tub, they seem to experience stronger contractions and many begin bargaining with me to get back in the water. That's what tells me it really works. I've even delivered many babies underwater that weren't planned waterbirths. The moms just got so comfortable, they didn't want to move."

What **Women** *Say About Laboring in Water and Waterbirth*

Jessica Kosa, who decided to have a waterbirth for the delivery of her second baby, at home

Why Did You Decide to Use Water Immersion?
"I am a huge wimp about pain, I hate pain, and had heard good things about both water and hypnosis during child-

birth, so in addition to water immersion, I took a childbirth preparation class that focused on deep relaxation, and I listened to the guided relaxation tapes often during my last trimester. I have chronic lower back pain, and believed that being in the water, with the weight off my back, would be helpful. I had labored in the bath for a bit during my first birth and liked it, so I expected that a full-sized tub would be even better."

Was Water Immersion What You Expected?

"Yes! I loved getting into the water when I was in active labor. I did not get in until late, but once I was in, I was very comfortable and decided to deliver in water."

Did Water Immersion Provide Pain Relief?

"I never had overwhelming pain. (The pain level, if I had it today, would probably be managed with a big dose of ibuprofen and rest.) I can't say how much of that was due to the water (as opposed to good positioning of the baby, relaxing home environment), but I am sure that the pushing stage was far more comfortable because I could just allow my body to find the best position without having to support weight. This birth was actually less painful than my first (despite the epidural the first time around), which I attribute partly to being a second-timer and partly to being very relaxed."

Would You Use Water Immersion Again?
"Absolutely."

Do You Think the Relief of Your Pain Impacted Your Satisfaction with Your Birth?

"Having good pain management was important for me, and definitely made the experience a completely happy memory for me. I was not pushed to my limit in pain tolerance, and I'm just as glad about that. I don't need to hurt to know I've given birth!"

Jennifer Howe, who used water immersion during labor for the birth of her second baby

Was Water Immersion What You Expected?

"I was very surprised that I actually did not like the tub. I couldn't get in a comfortable position and because my baby was born in August, the temperature of the water felt too hot to me."

Did Water Immersion Provide Pain Relief?

"The contractions did feel less intense, but because I was not comfortable in the tub—for the reasons mentioned above—I decided to get out. I did decide to use the tub after the baby was born, and found it very soothing."

Did You Use Any Other Comfort Measures or Pain-Relief Interventions?

"I liked the birth ball and did not use any form of medical pain relief."

Would You Use Water Immersion Again? Would You Recommend Other Women Use It?

"I might try it again for another birth, and I would recommend other women try it because I think my experience was the exception. I have heard that many other women have found it to be amazing during their labor and delivery."

Do You Think the Relief of Your Pain Impacted Your Satisfaction with Your Birth?

"I can't really say that the tub played a huge role in pain relief for me. I don't see the pain as getting in the way of the level of satisfaction I felt toward my birth experience. What I found most difficult was the length of the labor because I felt very tired and fatigued, but compared to my first baby's birth, a cesarean delivery, this birth was the most amazing and satisfying experience."

Resources

> www.waterbirth.org
> *Gentle Birth Choices,* 3rd ed., by Barbara Harper, R.N.
> (Rochester, VT: Healing Arts Press, 2005).

HYPNOTHERAPY—CHANGING YOUR *MIND* ABOUT LABOR PAIN

What It Is and What It Does

Hypnosis has been used for centuries as a pain-management technique, but even today it is still regarded as a kind of mystery by many people. Although techniques based on hypnosis have become more mainstream, misunderstandings about exactly what it is and how it works still exist. Hypnosis involves learning how to deeply relax both your body and mind through focused concentration. This state of concentration allows you to become more accepting of suggestions that can help you change your perceptions and your behaviors.

Hypnotherapy is the use of hypnosis to treat or alter a range of medical and nonmedical conditions and situations, including pain management in childbirth. The use of hypnotherapy as an approach to pain management during labor and birth has gained popularity in the last several years. Unlike most other CAM approaches, the philosophy of many programs that teach hypnosis for use during childbirth is that labor and birth do not have to be painful. Instructors (and users) of various hypnotic techniques suggest that hypnosis can be used effectively to reduce or eliminate fear and anxiety as well as pain and discomfort during childbirth. Whether hypnosis is seen as a pain-management tool or a pain-prevention tool, many women who choose hypnosis regard this technique as an effective and powerful approach to a comfortable—even pain-free—childbirth.

> **DID YOU KNOW?** *There is now a growing number of organizations throughout the country that specialize in teaching hypnotherapy as the primary or exclusive pain-management technique during childbirth.*

Hypnosis used for the purpose of pain management in childbirth is typically a technique women learn to do for themselves, not something done to them. This self-hypnosis is done using a variety of tools, including reading books, listening to tapes, taking sessions with a hypnotherapist, and practicing key words and phrases—known as hypnosis scripts—throughout the pregnancy.

A hypnotherapist typically teaches women the skill of self-hypnosis as a tool to use on their own, and often does not actually attend the labor and birth. Some programs, however, also have doulas who are trained in hypnotherapy available for support during childbirth.

Hypnotherapy for childbirth can be thought of as a kind of reconditioning of your expectations and perceptions about birth. Some have referred to the use of hypnosis for pain management during childbirth as an unlearning of negative expectations and messages women may hold toward the experience of childbirth. During a hypnotic state, these negative messages are replaced with positive ideas and images about what to expect during labor and birth. The theory is, when women expect birth to be a positive experience, free of fear and tension, their bodies will respond by relaxing and allowing birth to take place more easily.

DID YOU KNOW? *Stress hormones called catecholamines are released into your body when you experience or feel threatened by a stressful event. One of the goals of hypnosis is to reduce the flow of these stress hormones to allow your body (and mind) to relax and birth more easily.*

How It Is Done and How It Feels
Exactly how you use hypnosis during childbirth will depend largely on the philosophy of the individual or program you have chosen. Typically, there is a specific number of sessions spent with a hypnotherapist or instructor who teaches you how to use various relaxation techniques. These techniques may include deep-breathing exercises, visualization and guided imagery, or repetition of messages to yourself. Often the hypnotherapist provides tapes or CDs for you to listen to and practice with on your own or with your partner. These tapes or CDs can be used at the hospital or birth center throughout labor and birth. Some women may choose to have a doula who is trained in hypnotherapy for support during the labor and birth, but others simply use the techniques they have learned during pregnancy along with the support of their partner.

The sensations felt during hypnosis are different for everyone. Some people experience a light, floating sensation, while others describe a deep state of calm relaxation. In a state of hypnosis you continue to feel highly aware of and in control of yourself and your environment.

The type of support needed by the laboring mother who uses hypnosis can be quite different from the support typically needed by most other laboring women. Since hypnosis aims to change your perceptions of the sensations of childbirth, it involves using entirely different words to describe labor pain. Contractions are often referred to as rushes or surges, in an attempt to divert the mind's attention from a negative association with the physical experience of contractions during labor.

> The use of specific words is key to hypnosis. Women are typically discouraged from using any language that has a negative emotional association. For instance, the chapter in this book called "Your Labor Pain" might instead be called "Your Labor Sensations" if written by a hypnotherapist.

If nurses and caregivers are unaware of the specific needs of a laboring woman using hypnosis, the supportive statements typically used to help laboring women ("This is hard work, but you're doing great," or "The pain will pass") may actually break her concentration.

Some hypnosis birth programs provide a user-friendly information sheet that the mom hands to her nurses and physicians upon her arrival to the maternity unit. This sheet lets the staff know that the mom will be using hypnosis and tells them what words and hypnotic cues the mom (and partner) will be using, so that they can better assist her during labor and birth.

> **DID YOU KNOW?** *Most hypnosis techniques used during childbirth are based on the idea that when you change your **expectation** of childbirth, you can change your **experience** of childbirth.*

Reasons You May Choose to Use Hypnosis for Pain Relief

- You prefer to use no medication.
- You want to avoid your pain, reduce your pain, or have an effective coping tool to deal with your labor pain.
- You want to give birth in a quiet and calm setting in which you are able to control your own sensations.

Your Partner's Role During Hypnotherapy

In most childbirth hypnosis programs the partner plays a vital role in the birth experience. Often your partner is taught how to help you use your self-hypnosis material during labor and delivery. Your partner's role may be to assist you via verbal or physical cues meant to help keep you focused or deepen your hypnotic state.

Potential Benefits of Hypnotherapy

- Many women have found that hypnosis allowed them to experience sensations of pressure rather than pain throughout labor and delivery.
- Women using hypnosis who experienced sensations of pain during childbirth reported that hypnosis helped them cope with their discomfort.
- Many hypnotherapy methods also allow for the use of medical pain relief if you so desire.
- The use of self-hypnosis can help you deal with many of the discomforts associated with pregnancy—sleep disturbances, nausea, headache, backache, and tension— even before you need it in the delivery room.
- The use of self-hypnosis for pain management can also help you cope with postdelivery pain and discomfort.

Potential Limitations of Hypnotherapy

- Learning self-hypnosis involves preparation and the expense of taking a course or hiring a hypnotherapist.
- Success requires commitment and the ability to practice consistently for several weeks or months prior to giving birth.
- Your caregivers at the hospital or birthing center will need special instruction to ensure they understand and can accommodate your specific needs.

Hypnosis Concerns and Controversies

No medical concerns or controversies currently exist regarding the use of hypnosis during childbirth. Hypnosis is considered a highly safe method to use during childbirth.

> **RESEARCH SAYS:** *In the most comprehensive review of literature on the use of hypnosis for pain relief during childbirth, studies involving over eight thousand women were evaluated and it was shown that women who used hypnosis during childbirth rated their pain as less severe than women who did not. The review also concluded that hypnosis reduces the need for pain-relief medications during childbirth.*[17]

A Caregiver's Perspective

Kerry Tuschhoff, a certified hypnosis instructor, certified hypnotherapist, and doula, founder of Hypnobabies Network, a program that teaches hypnosis to expecting moms

"Hypnosis literally re-creates your inner belief systems about childbirth, then programs your belief systems to have only positive expectations for labor. Hypnosis for childbirth is like a software for your mind. Does it take more of a time commitment to practice childbirth hypnosis than other methods?

Probably so, since you will need to hear your hypnotic suggestions every day to make sure your inner mind continues its computer reprogramming. This, however, is the easiest thing that you will do as you prepare for your baby's birth, easier than picking out your new baby's car seat!

"In my experience, observing my own students as they give birth, and interviewing them afterward, women are very in tune with their babies and their own bodies, completely aware of everything that is going on inside and around them, yet their inner focus is on relaxation and complete physical comfort."

What Women *Say About Hypnosis*

Jennie Reiff, who used hypnosis during the birth of her first baby

Why Did You Decide to Use Hypnosis?
"When I first found out I was pregnant, I never even considered a natural birth. I wanted as many drugs as they could give me, so I would not feel the pain. But, when I was about four months pregnant, I saw a story about hypnosis on the news that claimed that women could have a natural, pain-free birth. I was skeptical but my husband and I decided to look into it. As we learned more, we decided it was worth a try. I figured, as long as I could have a pain-free birth, I might as well have it without drugs if possible. I spoke to my obstetrician about our interest in hypnosis and she referred us to an instructor who had worked with another patient of hers. (My obstetrician also added she had been amazed by that patient's delivery.) So we took the recommendation and proceeded from there."

Did Hypnosis Provide Pain Relief?
"I can't say for sure if hypnosis provided pain relief, because I never felt any labor pain to be relieved of. So, I have to imagine that the technique provided tremendous pain relief. My

whole labor lasted five and a half hours. I felt discomfort and pressure but nothing unbearable. Once I started pushing, I felt no more discomfort at all. I felt my son being born, but felt absolutely no pain, even though I tore a little. I never felt the 'ring of fire' that people talked about. I didn't even bother using any pain medication, not even the Midol the hospital offered, after I gave birth."

How Was Your Partner Involved?

"My husband attended all of the classes and practiced scripts [written material with cue words and phrases used for self-hypnosis] with me whenever they were scheduled. He helped write our birth plan and wanted to be as involved in the birth as possible. He read me a script early in my labor and encouraged me throughout."

Would You Use Hypnosis Again and Recommend It to Other Women?

"I would absolutely use hypnosis again. It worked so perfectly, I can't imagine using anything else. When I went in for my six-week follow-up appointment, the obstetrician who delivered my baby (who was not my regular obstetrician) said, 'You're the one who did the hypnosis. That was the most amazing birth I have ever seen.' She told me she called her own mother to tell her about it!"

Sheila Faris-Penn, who used hypnosis during the birth of her first baby

Why Did You Decide to Use Hypnosis?

"The idea of a drug-free birth really appealed to me and my husband, but I had always thought that you just went without, and suffered. I was planning to try going without drugs, but not be 'heroic' if I was in too much pain. I am also a serious 'pain-wuss' so I was not sure I would be able to give birth without medication."

Did Hypnosis Provide Pain Relief?

"Other than some discomfort, I really had no trouble. When my water broke I began listening to my hypnosis CD, and felt no pain for several hours. Then my cat jumped into my lap and landed, hard, in the middle of my belly, bringing me out of hypnosis. That's when I discovered how well the hypnosis had been working! I managed to get back into hypnosis. From that point on all I felt was discomfort. I used no other comfort measures or pain-relief interventions."

Did the Relief of Your Pain Impact Your Level of Satisfaction with Your Birth?

"Yes, I think the relative lack of pain was a major factor in how wonderful my birth experience was. There really wasn't anything more than discomfort and that was worth it. A drug-free birth was a gift I gave to my son and I wouldn't have it any other way; he was so alert when he was born. It was amazing."

Kimberly Milo, a mother of two whose babies were born with the use of hypnosis

Why Did You Decide to Use Hypnosis?

"I wanted a method that made sense with my spiritual and physical philosophy toward birth. I did not even know these techniques existed and through my prenatal yoga instructor, I discovered them. Hypnosis fit exactly with what I was looking for to ease my nervousness and fear about birthing."

Did Hypnosis Provide Pain Relief?

"The hypnosis program I used absolutely provided pain relief. I knew exactly what to do through the whole process, as I had practiced so consistently and thoroughly for months. At one point, I was actually smiling through a birthing wave as I realized my daughter was closer to being in my arms. I also used the technique after delivery when I was given Pitocin to help my uterus contract."

Did the Relief of Your Pain Impact Your Level of Satisfaction with Your Birth?

"Absolutely. When I think of the birth of both of my babies, I don't have fear or anxiety. In fact, I am excited for the next one and my youngest is only nine and a half weeks old. Using hypnosis was easier the second time because I knew what to expect. My main reason for searching for an alternative birth method was that I needed something that would put my mind at ease as much as possible, whether I ended up going drug-free or not. Hypnosis tamed that fear and provided a deep joy and peace instead."

Kimberly Pearson, who used hypnosis during the birth of her first baby

Why Did You Decide to Use Hypnosis?

"I had scoliosis surgery as a teenager, and my obstetrician told me I would not be able to use an epidural, so I looked into other methods of pain relief. I had heard of hypnosis but did not know anything about it. At a hospital open house one of the hypnosis instructors was there, and when I spoke with her I became interested in learning more. I attended the hypnosis courses and thought, Why would I do it any other way?"

Did Hypnosis Provide Pain Relief?

"I had absolutely no pain the entire time. I felt pressure, but it was completely manageable. I felt the sensation that my skin was stretching when the baby was crowning, but there was no pain involved, even during the birth of the baby. It worked better than I had hoped."

How Was Your Partner Involved?

"He took classes and helped me practice. During labor he walked me through contractions and helped me focus. We also had a doula who was a hypnosis instructor. She was with me throughout the more active part of my [long] labor."

Did the Relief of Your Pain Impact Your Level of Satisfaction with Your Birth?

"Yes, less pain absolutely makes for a more satisfying birth experience for me. I was thrilled with the whole experience. It was totally pleasant. I could feel everything I wanted to feel. I could get up and walk around. My son's birth was an absolutely incredible experience!"

Resources

Hypnobabies Network
Kerry Tuschhoff, HCHI, CHt
71801 Katella Avenue, Suite 241
Stanton, CA 90680
www.hypnobabies.com

Or, use your favorite Internet search engine and type in the words *hypnosis during childbirth* to locate additional organizations and resources.

ACUPUNCTURE DURING CHILDBIRTH

What It Is and What It Does
Acupuncture is an ancient Chinese therapeutic technique in which a trained practitioner inserts very thin, long metal needles just under your skin at different points on your body. The acupuncture technique is based on the concept that there is an energy flow throughout the body called chi. When this energy flow is disrupted in some way, the strategic placement of the acupuncture needles can restore its balance, resulting in improved health or pain relief.

Acupuncture is most commonly used in the United States by people seeking relief for chronic pain; the use of acupuncture for pain relief during childbirth is still rare in this country, but has gained popularity over the last twenty years. Some hospitals and birth centers now allow acupuncture to be used when women hire their own acupuncturist to attend their birth.

How acupuncture actually works is unclear. One theory suggests it stimulates the release of certain chemicals or hormones, called endorphins—which act as pain relievers—into your muscles, spinal cord, and brain. The body's production of these natural pain relievers (which are chemically similar to narcotics) can change your perception of pain, may boost your body's own natural healing abilities, and may promote feelings of physical and emotional well-being.

How It Is Done and How It Feels

Acupuncture needles for labor-pain relief are generally placed in the arms and legs, or in the ear area. Other body points used during labor include your hands, ankles, and lower back. Although the sensation of receiving acupuncture is different for everyone, most people feel no pain or minimal pain when the needles are inserted into their skin. Once the needles are in place, the acupuncturist may twist them or apply a weak electrical current to increase the energy flow. The needles typically remain in place for fifteen to forty minutes, depending on the condition or source of pain that is being treated. Some people report feeling energized after an acupuncture treatment, and others find they experience a sense of relaxation afterward.

Why You May Choose Acupuncture

Women who choose acupuncture generally want to avoid the use of medications during childbirth. Often women who prefer acupuncture are already using alternative medicine in other aspects of their health care, including their prenatal care. Even if you have never used acupuncture, however, it may be a method of pain reduction and relaxation during childbirth that interests you.

DID YOU KNOW? *Some acupuncturists will use a technique called* moxibustion *to turn a breech baby. This technique is highly successful and works on approximately 80 percent of women who try it. Moxibustion involves burning certain herbs around specific sites on the mom's feet. The moxa plant is placed as close as possible to the outside of the little toe and directed at the point just above the toenail for about twenty minutes. Moxibustion works by stimulating fetal movement, so the baby actually turns itself, usually within six to eight hours of treatment.*[18]

When Can You Use Acupuncture?

According to Valerie Hobbs, a licensed acupuncturist and associate professor at Southwest Acupuncture College, "Promoting wellness by preparing your body through the use of acupuncture treatments before childbirth, throughout your pregnancy, is one of the primary ways in which you can maximize the chances that any pain you experience will be minimized, because the acupuncture balances the entire system. In addition, acupuncture is used to directly relieve pain during childbirth."

Once your labor begins, it is to your advantage to begin acupuncture treatments in early labor, before the pain intensifies. If you begin the release of your body's natural painkilling chemicals, endorphins, sooner rather than later, you may be able to stay ahead of your pain as your contractions get stronger.

Your Partner's Role During Your Acupuncture Treatment

Your partner can help you in the same way he would if you were using any other method of pain relief: by providing you with comfort and emotional support throughout labor and birth.

Potential Benefits of Acupuncture

- Acupuncture is especially beneficial when used for painful "back labor."
- There are no side effects.
- You can combine acupuncture with the use of other pain-relief methods, including epidurals and other pain-relief medications.

Potential Limitations of Acupuncture

- You need an acupuncturist available to you at your place of birth.
- Acupuncture may not provide you with enough pain relief.

Potential Side Effects of Acupuncture

- Fainting upon needle insertion is the most common side effect, although this rarely happens.
- Stimulating certain acupuncture points (lower abdomen and lower back) could stimulate uterine contractions and induce premature labor.
- Slight bruising can occur at the acupuncture site.

Conditions or Situations That Would Prevent You from Using Acupuncture

- If you are on anticoagulant drugs and bleed easily, you should consult your physician before using acupuncture.
- If you have multiple health problems, you may wish to consult your physician while seeking acupuncture care.

RESEARCH SAYS: *In a review of studies conducted on the effectiveness of complementary and alternative therapies for pain management during childbirth, a study involving one hundred women who used acupuncture demonstrated a decreased need for pain relief and concluded, "Acupuncture (and hypnosis) may be beneficial for the management of pain during labor."*[19]

A Caregiver's Perspective

Marsha Connor, R.N., Oriental Medical Doctor, a licensed acupuncturist, who routinely uses acupuncture on women during childbirth

"In my experience, women who use acupuncture during childbirth are usually well educated and interested in having a drug-free birth for the health of their baby and themselves. They find that the acupuncture is very helpful for relaxation and useful in making the labor contractions more effective and less painful."

Resources
Most (but not all) states provide licensure. To find a certified acupuncturist in your community or to learn more:

National Commission for Certification of
Acupuncture and Oriental Medicine
www.nccaom.org

American Association of Oriental Medicine
P.O. Box 162340
Sacramento, CA 95816
www.aaom.org

National Center for Complementary and Alternative
Medicine
National Institutes of Health
Bethesda, MD 20892
www.nccam.nih.gov

Labor Support

What It Is and What It Does
Labor support is the very basic concept of one-on-one care
provided to you from the beginning of your labor until the
birth of the baby. This "new" approach is centuries old, but is
just beginning to pick up momentum as a popular birth option.
The person who is most likely to provide such support today is
a doula or midwife.

In a typical maternity unit, physicians, nurses, and, in some
hospitals, midwives, will attend to your care. However, in a
hospital setting, staff members have additional responsibilities
and are typically caring for several patients at one time, which
means they are unable to devote all of their time specifically
to you while you labor. In addition, the person who spends
the most time with you during labor—the labor and delivery
nurse—no matter how caring and competent, is almost always
someone you have never met before, and the nurses caring for
you during labor may change as their shifts change throughout
the day.

By contrast, your labor support person is someone with
whom you are familiar, who will provide constant companionship to you throughout your entire childbirth experience. Labor
support consists of emotional support and encouragement for
you (and your partner), making you aware of what is happening to you and your baby during the process of labor and birth,
and implementing comfort measures and pain-management
strategies according to your own preferences. Labor support
ensures that, in addition to the staff responsible for your care at

the hospital, you will be given constant attention by one person throughout your labor and birth.

> **DID YOU KNOW?** *The majority of women who receive continuous labor support prefer this type of care and would ask for it again. Labor-support services are increasing to meet growing demand, as more women are learning about the benefits of having a professional labor-support person during childbirth. One recent survey estimated that 5 percent of the respondents had used the services of a doula during childbirth. According to the American College of Nurse Midwives, approximately 10 percent of births involve the care of a midwife.*

How It Is Done and How It Feels

Most often you will have met with your doula or midwife prior to your due date. During this introductory meeting, she may provide details about what to expect during labor and birth and will listen to your own preferences for the type of birth you desire and what kind of comfort measures or pain-relief methods you would like to use once labor begins.

Typically, you will call your doula or midwife when you think labor has begun. She may just stay in touch, checking with you by phone, until your labor progresses, or she may come to your home until you are ready to go to the hospital. Or, your doula or midwife may arrange to join you when you first arrive on the maternity unit. Some prefer to arrive once you have progressed to active labor. Regardless of when your doula or midwife arrives, you will usually benefit from her services as soon she joins you.

Once your labor-support person arrives at your home or place of birth, depending on where you are and how you are progressing, she may begin by giving you a massage, helping you to use a birth ball, or encouraging you to use the bath or shower or to walk around if you are comfortable enough to do so. Some bring tapes with soothing sounds, affirmative messages, or music. Most likely, you will have already decided ahead of time what you would like her to bring as comfort measures during labor.

The emotional support and advice from a birthing expert may help you feel more in control and less overwhelmed, especially if this is your first childbirth. Your doula or midwife can provide verbal support, help you time your contractions, and help you communicate with those on the hospital staff who are caring for you. You may feel physically pampered by the extra comforts provided in the form of massage, music, aromatherapy, and any other creature comforts she knows will make your birth easier.

You should feel well informed about what to expect as your labor progresses and your labor-support person will know how to encourage your efforts and provide empathy, support, and assistance if you reach a point where you feel you are running out of steam.

Your doula or midwife will have expertise in the use of movement and positioning and can help you find the best possible position for your own comfort level. She will know when it might be timely for you to try using the various techniques available to you in your specific birth setting, that is, when it's best to try the shower or bath, when to get up and walk around, and when (and how) to reposition yourself in bed.

Why You Would Choose to Use Labor Support

- You want constant, one-on-one expertise and a more personalized level of care during your labor and birth.
- You are concerned your partner might be overwhelmed and unable to provide the level of support and encouragement a professional can offer.
- Your previous birth experience was unsatisfactory, and

you want someone there to help you have a better birth experience.

- You do not want to use medical pain relief and would like labor support to help you successfully use nonmedical pain-management techniques.
- You plan to use pain relief whenever you feel you need to but would like the care and comfort a professional labor-support person offers throughout the entire birth experience.

Your Partner's Role

Your partner will still play an important role, of course, as your key support person, but will probably be relieved to have someone who understands what to expect, knows how to meet your very specific needs during labor, and can give both of you advice. Partners can often feel frustrated or overwhelmed while their loved one is in labor. The presence of a skilled labor-support person can provide reassurance and encouragement to your partner, who may at various points in your labor feel frustrated or unable to offer the help you may need.

Another clear advantage to your partner of having a labor-support person present is that he can take a break or get some rest without feeling like he's abandoning you. He won't be able to do this once you're both home with your new baby, so make sure he understands this is a very time-limited perk!

Potential Benefits of Labor Support

- Improves overall satisfaction with childbirth experience.
- May enhance your feelings of control and competence during labor and birth.
- May help reduce your fear and anxiety level by having someone knowledgeable and supportive throughout your labor and birth.
- May reduce your use of pain medication.
- No known risks.

Potential Limitations of Labor Support

- Generally, you will have to pay for your own labor-support person, because the hospital or insurance company typically does not. It is worth asking your insurer, however, whether it will cover some or all of the costs.

RESEARCH SAYS: *In the study "Continuous Support for Women during Childbirth," fifteen trials, which included thirteen thousand women, were reviewed to assess the effects on mothers and their babies of continuous one-on-one labor support. The results: "Women who had continuous labor support were less likely to use analgesia [pain-relief medication], have an operative birth [cesarean, forceps, or vacuum extraction] or report dissatisfaction with their childbirth experiences." The benefits were shown to be greater when the labor-support person was not a member of the hospital staff, when labor support was initiated in early labor, and when the birth took place in settings where epidurals were not routinely available. The study concluded: "All women should have support throughout labor and birth."[20]*

In another study, cesarean section rates were compared between two groups of laboring women, those who had continuous labor support by nurses employed by the hospitals and those who did not. The rates of cesarean delivery were almost identical. However, the women who had the continuous labor-support preferred this type of care and 46 percent of the women who were in the group without the labor support expressed a desire to have continuous labor support in future childbirth experiences.[21]

A Caregiver's Perspective

Jane Look, a certified childbirth doula in Boston, Massachusetts

"Many families tell me that the support of a skilled doula is worth her weight in gold. The most common comment is that they couldn't have done it without her. As doulas, we know these families could have birthed without us. We also know that they would not have had someone, every moment, of every hour, there to support them through one of the most amazing times of their lives."

Resources

DONA International
P.O. Box 626
Jasper, IN 47547
www.DONA.org

Childbirth and Postpartum Professional Association (CAPPA)
P.O. Box 491448
Lawrenceville, GA 30049
www.CAPPA.net

Association of Labor Assistants and Childbirth Educators (ALACE)
P.O. Box 390436
Cambridge, MA 02139
www.alace.org

If you are interested in learning more about labor support, read:

The Birth Partner: Everything You Need to Know to Help a Woman Through Childbirth, 2nd ed., by Penny Simkin (Boston: The Harvard Common Press, 2001).

AROMATHERAPY

What It Is and What It Does
Aromatherapy is the use of essential oils taken from the roots, leaves, or blossoms of certain plants for the purpose of

healing and promoting a sense of calm and relaxation. Aromatherapy is fairly new to the maternity unit but appears to be gaining popularity as a comfort measure for laboring women.

How It Is Done and How It Feels

Aromatherapy is applied primarily in two ways. Oil or lotion can be applied to your skin via massage, or you can inhale the fragrance of various essential oils in a number of different ways. The essential oil may be applied to a small slip of paper, called a taper, which is then attached to your hospital gown or clothing, close enough to your face for you to breathe in, or it may be placed in a diffuser, which uses a fan to disperse the fragrance throughout your room.

Some essential oils are thought to help reduce pain by enhancing relaxation. The pleasant, soothing qualities of certain fragrances may trigger a positive emotional response that may help you relax. Even if no direct pain relief is experienced, aromatherapy may help to reduce your anxiety level and help you cope better throughout your labor. Exactly how these aromas may affect your health and emotional state is not fully understood. In addition, there is not a lot of information on how these essential oils interact with conventional medicine. It is recommended that you check with your physician or midwife before using any essential oils during pregnancy and childbirth. There is limited research on the use of aromatherapy during childbirth, but many claims are made to the healing and soothing powers of aromatherapy in general.

Below we have provided a list of the essential oils commonly used during childbirth and the healing properties associated with each.

The Essential Oils Typically Used During Childbirth

Lavender is one of the most popular essential oils and is thought to reduce anxiety and produce feelings of relaxation.

Frankincense is thought to promote feelings of calm and to help laboring women breathe more slowly and deeply. Frankincense oil is used specifically for massage during childbirth.

Bergamot is often used for patients who are experiencing anxiety. For pain relief, bergamot must be massaged into your body, at or near the source of your pain—typically abdomen or lower back.

Clary sage is believed to help stimulate the uterus, induce labor, strengthen contractions, and have pain-relieving qualities. It can sometimes have a euphoric effect. Clary sage oil should be avoided during pregnancy because it can be toxic if applied in high doses. This oil should be used to stimulate contractions only under the close supervision of medical personnel trained in aromatherapy.

Peppermint is thought to have antiseptic (germ-killing) properties. When inhaled, it may reduce nausea and vomiting in some laboring women.

Rose oil is thought to be useful in reducing anxiety during labor.

Neroli is thought to reduce fear, anxiety, and tension during labor.

Roman chamomile is used during labor when the patient needs rest. It has a calming and relaxing effect. It can be useful to promote sleep, especially in women who experience a particularly long and difficult early labor.

When Can You Use Aromatherapy?

You can use aromatherapy throughout labor, until just prior to delivery. Since there is currently no research available on the safety of diffusing essential oils around newborns, just as a precautionary measure it is best to stop diffusing oils an hour before delivery.

You should choose which fragrances you prefer before

your labor begins, to avoid the use of fragrances you find undesirable. In using essential oils, less is better; do not diffuse the oils for more than fifteen minutes each hour. If you do not have a diffuser, you can place a drop of essential oil on a tissue and place the tissue in your pillowcase. If you have an epidural at any point during labor, the use of essential oils associated with lowering blood pressure, including lavender, clary sage, lemon, marjoram, and ylang-ylang, is not recommended.

Your Partner's Role

- Your partner's key role in the use of essential oils is as masseur. He can use the essential oils you have chosen to massage you during labor. When essential oils are massaged into the skin, they must be diluted in a carrier oil such as sweet almond oil or olive oil. When mixing essential oils for massage, use only one to three drops of the desired essential oil in five milliliters (one teaspoon) of a carrier oil. Roll the bottle containing the oils vigorously between your hands to mix. Do not shake the bottle. One teaspoon of the massage oil mixture is enough for a whole-body massage.
- If you don't find massage soothing, your partner can spritz the fragrance in the air around you using a spray bottle containing your essential oils. (When spritzing essential oils, mix four to five drops of essential oil in one pint of distilled water.)
- Your partner can hold a handkerchief or cloth that has been sprayed or rubbed with the aromatherapy oil for you to smell whenever you like.

Potential Benefits of Aromatherapy

- Your body may respond to the calming and relaxing qualities of the essential oils.

- Aromatherapy may provide a distraction from your discomfort.
- Certain essential oils, such as peppermint, may help alleviate nausea.
- You may feel soothed by the pleasant fragrances.
- Aromatherapy can be used with any form of pain management you choose.

Potential Limitations of Aromatherapy

- You should only use 100 percent pure therapeutic essential oils. It is thought that the pure essential oils possess the properties that are responsible for the healing and soothing effects of aromatherapy.
- Since your sense of smell may be heightened during pregnancy, certain essential oils may make you feel nauseous.
- You may have an allergic reaction to a particular aromatherapy mixture.
- You should always consult with your caregiver before using any essential oils during pregnancy and childbirth.

RESEARCH SAYS: *A study of over eight thousand women who used aromatherapy in the maternity unit to relieve anxiety, pain, nausea, and vomiting, or to strengthen contractions, reported that the majority of these women found it helpful during labor.*[22]

A Caregiver's Bath Recipe Used for Aromatherapy During Childbirth

Nancy Wiand, a clinical nurse specialist who has developed one of the few aromatherapy programs in the country for laboring women, at Robinson Memorial Hospital in Ravenna, Ohio

"I recommend the following bath blend using lavender essential oil.

Step one: Fill tub before adding oils, or they will evaporate too quickly.

Step two: Add an ingredient that will help your essential oil mix with your bath water, known as a dispersal agent. This can be milk or cream, about one teaspoon for a normal-sized bathtub.

Step three: Add approximately five to ten drops of the lavender essential oil and swish around the water in the tub to mix the various ingredients.

Step four: Soak and relax. If the lavender is really working for you, spritz some of the solution on a cloth handkerchief and take it 'to go' to your hospital or birthing center.

Tip: Hang on to this bath-blend recipe to use when you return home with your baby. You're going to need to take some precious time for yourself and you can enjoy this again.

"Women with allergies are advised to do a skin test before using essential oils in a bath. To do this, dilute six drops of the desired essential oil in one teaspoon of a carrier oil (such as almond oil or olive oil). Place a drop on the inner forearm, cover with a bandage for twenty-four hours, then observe the site for any skin irritation. If there is no rash, that oil can be used in your bath."

Resources

> National Association for Holistic Aromatherapy
> 3327 W. Indian Trail Road PMB 144
> Spokane, WA 99208
> www.naha.org

Read:
> *Clinical Aromatherapy for Pregnancy and Childbirth,* 2nd ed., by
> Denise Tiran (London: Churchill Livingstone, 2000).

STERILE WATER PAPULES

What They Are and What They Do
Sterile water papules are injections of sterile water into the skin
of your lower back. This technique is used almost exclusively to
relieve painful back labor. The idea behind this type of treatment is that the labor-pain messages your brain is receiving will
be overridden by the new pain messages of the sterile water injections, essentially tricking your brain into feeling the other
(less painful) stimulation of the injections rather than the more
intense pain of your contractions. The pain relief can take place
within minutes of the injections.

DID YOU KNOW? *It is estimated that approximately 30
percent of women experience back labor during childbirth.*[23]

How It Is Done and How It Feels
Your nurse or midwife will have you get into a comfortable
position, lying down on your side or bending over the bed.
The skin on your lower back is cleaned with an alcohol swab.
A tiny amount of sterile water is injected just under the skin
in four places at the base of the spine. The injections will cause

an intense burning feeling, much like a bee sting, but the pain only lasts about thirty to sixty seconds. When the pain from the injection is gone, you will often have significant relief of your back pain by the time the next contraction arrives. Some women report that they experience relief from their back pain for up to two hours after the sterile water injections. Other women find that their pain persists in spite of the treatment.

Why You Would Choose Sterile Water Papules

- You are having extreme back pain during labor.
- You wish to avoid the use of medications during labor.

> *Do sterile water papule injections really provide pain relief?* Some research suggests that 70 to 90 percent of women who use this technique for relief of painful back labor experience pain relief for at least one hour after receiving the sterile water injections.[24]

When Can You Use Sterile Water Papules?

Since this treatment involves inflicting pain (briefly) to reduce pain (for an hour or more), the timing of its use depends entirely on how much pain you are experiencing. If, on a scale of one to ten, you are rating your pain high (typically seven or more), then you are more likely to benefit from this technique.

Your Partner's Role

Your partner can help you by holding your hands and comforting you during the injections, but he should not rub your back after the sterile water injections because doing so may reduce the effectiveness of the treatment.

Potential Benefits of Sterile Water Papules

- There are no known side effects other than the discomfort of the injections.
- This procedure is very quick and simple.
- This procedure uses no medication.
- This technique can be used in addition to IV medications.

Potential Limitations of Sterile Water Papules

- Many labor units do not use this technique.
- The injections themselves are quite painful. However, they should be far less painful than back labor.
- This pain-relief method does not relieve abdominal labor pain.

RESEARCH SAYS: *In one study on the effectiveness of the use of sterile water papules, eighty-three women with low back pain at the beginning of labor were given sterile water injections. There was "instant and complete relief of low back pain in all but 6 women, this effect lasting in many cases as long as 3 hours," after which they could receive additional injections. "Half of the women required no further analgesia during the first stage of labor." Of the eighty-three women who had the sterile water papules, sixty-seven women said they would use them again for their next labor.*[25]

A Caregiver's Perspective

Jude Stensland, a nurse-midwife now in family practice, who used sterile water papules for years in her childbirth practice

"Sterile water papules have been one of my most effective tools for relieving the pain of back labor. I always tell women that the injections do sting fiercely for a minute, but then the back pain will usually be relieved. Most women are really surprised at the relief that follows the stinging."

Resources
You will need to check with your obstetrician or midwife to find out if sterile water papules are an option in your birth setting.

TRANSCUTANEOUS ELECTRICAL NERVE STIMULATION (TENS)—THE "ELECTRICAL MASSAGE"

What It Is and What It Does
Transcutaneous electrical nerve stimulation (TENS) is a device that emits electrical stimulation to specific nerves for the purpose of providing comfort or distraction from pain. This device is used to treat various types of pain and discomfort, including labor pain. The TENS is a small, handheld device about the size of a television remote control. Electrode pads connected by wires to the device are on or near the site of pain. These pads can deliver two different types of electrical stimulation: a "burst" type of stimulation, typically used for chronic or more moderate pain, and a more constant stimulation, used for acute, short-lived pain, like the pain of contractions.

TENS sends electrical stimulation to your nerves, which blocks labor-pain signals to the brain and may also stimulate your body's production of endorphins, natural painkillers. The way in which TENS affects your pain level is similar to how pain relief is achieved through the use of sterile water papules, described in pages 191–194 in this chapter.

How It Is Done and How It Feels
You operate the TENS device. When it is turned on it will deliver mild electrical impulses to the area under the electrodes. The electrical stimulation may feel like a buzzing or tingling

sensation. Some women report that TENS reduces their pain and that the distraction makes coping with contractions more tolerable. Others report that the use of TENS makes no difference at all in their comfort level. It may be a good technique to try if you do not want an epidural or other pain-relief medication. Or you may choose to use TENS for relief in early labor to delay your use of an epidural or other pain-relief medications.

When Can You Use TENS?

It can take up to thirty minutes before you may feel the effects of TENS. For best results, TENS should be used in early labor. Women in active labor report that TENS does not provide adequate pain relief. TENS is available only by prescription from your physician, and arrangements should be made for its use prior to your arrival in the maternity unit.

Your Partner's Role

Your partner can continue to provide emotional support to you while you are using the TENS machine. You and your caregiver will attend to adjusting the placement of the electrode pads and to the settings on the TENS machine.

Potential Benefits of TENS

- TENS can be used with other pain-relief interventions.
- TENS may help you delay or avoid the use of medications.
- You are able to control the device and the amount of electrical stimulation you receive.

Potential Limitations of TENS

- Not all hospital labor units offer TENS.
- TENS does not always provide relief, even in early labor.
- Two percent of patients may have an allergic-type skin reaction to the gel, tape, or electrode material.

> **RESEARCH SAYS:** *The research done on the use of TENS during labor is contradictory. One study, which examined the effectiveness of TENS used for pain relief during labor, concluded that the majority of the respondents (72 percent of the first-time moms and 69 percent of the repeat moms) considered TENS effective for relief of their labor pain.*[26]
>
> *However, a separate clinical review concluded that the use of TENS does not relieve labor pain. In this review of studies involving 712 women, researchers stated there "was no compelling evidence for TENS having any analgesic effect during labor."*[27]

A Caregiver's Perspective

Margie Bissinger, a physical therapist in private practice who conducted a study on the effectiveness of TENS as a pain-management technique during childbirth and decided to use TENS for her own pain management during the birth of her first child

"The TENS really did help. My labor was induced and TENS definitely took the edge off of the pain for the first several hours of my early labor. I went on to have an epidural, which was wonderful, but TENS definitely helped me and has its place during early labor. Even though I used an epidural for my next two children, I still believe that TENS is great for women who do not want an epidural or are having a baby in a place where an epidural is not an option."

Resources

TENS devices are usually available in the hospital setting. You will need to speak with your physician in advance to order a TENS device before you get to the hospital or birth center.

THE BIRTH BALL

What It Is and What It Does

A birth ball is a large, air-filled vinyl ball similar to the kind you often find used in fitness centers or gymnasiums. It has traditionally been used by physical therapists for rehabilitation therapy, but has recently become popular for use during labor.

The birth ball is used to sit on during labor and allows you to rock and reposition your weight easily. The birth ball can help you get into more comfortable positions that you could not get into while in bed or sitting down. Sitting on the ball can also take some of the pressure off of your perineal (vaginal and rectal) area.

How It Is Done and How It Feels

A birth ball is unstable and rolly, so you may need someone to help you stay balanced while you sit or rock on it. Many women use the birth ball to "hug" by leaning over onto it, as if kneeling on all fours. By using the ball for this position there is less strain on your arms, hands, and knees. The ball can also be used for support while in the squatting position. When you are no longer comfortable enough to walk around, the birth ball can help keep you active during labor.

Repositioning with the help of the birth ball is more comfortable for some women than simply changing positions in bed or in a chair. The ball itself has some give to it and this helps provide a softer surface as you try to get into comfortable positions.

> The use of the birth ball does not eliminate your pain but it can enhance your ability to cope with your contractions.

When Can You Use the Birth Ball?

When you are in early labor at home the birth ball may help you feel more comfortable, and it can be brought with you to the birthing unit (or they may have their own). The birth ball can be used throughout labor, and even if you decide to have a light epidural, you may be able to continue using the ball in some hospitals, with assistance.

Your Partner's Role

- Your partner can "spot" you on the ball, providing assistance to prevent you from losing your balance.
- He can continue to massage you while you find a comfortable position on the ball.

Potential Benefits of the Birth Ball

- Use of the birth ball may increase your comfort and help you cope with labor pain.
- Use of the birth ball can encourage fetal descent and pelvic relaxation.
- There are no side effects.
- The birth ball is very simple to use.

Potential Limitations of the Birth Ball

- Not all hospital units provide them.
- The effects of certain pain-relief medications that may make you feel drowsy or unsteady may prevent you from using it.
- If you are allergic to latex, make certain the type of ball you have contains none.

A Caregiver's Perspective

Paulina Perez, R.N., a doula, childbirth educator, and author of several books on childbirth

"The use of the birth ball is so simple. Sitting on the rolling surface of the birth ball challenges the mother's body and the ball can be used in countless ways. The appropriate size of the birth ball is determined by the height of the woman using it. The round ball positions the mother's center of gravity over her base of support and activates the muscles of the feet, legs, hips, and spine in order to maintain the woman's balance. While sitting on the round ball, the woman's hips and knees should be bent at ninety-degree angles and her knees should be directly over her ankles.

"The size that seems to work best with laboring mothers is the sixty-five–centimeter (25½-inch) round ball. The ball should be inflated to the point that is slightly firm but still 'gives' and rolls easily. Most hospital maternity obstetric departments offer birth balls of different sizes and shapes so that the nurse, midwife, or labor assistant can choose the best ball for specific use in the individual woman's labor."

Resources
www.birthballs.com—Contains a gallery of photos and information on using birth balls in maternity care as well as information on where to order a birth ball.

READING
Birth Balls: The Physical Therapy Balls in Maternity Care, by Paulina Perez (Johnson, VT: Cutting Edge Press, 2000).

Seven

PAIN RELIEF FOR A CESAREAN DELIVERY—THE EPIDURAL, THE SPINAL, AND GENERAL ANESTHESIA

WHAT EXACTLY IS A CESAREAN DELIVERY?

A cesarean delivery is a surgical procedure in which an incision is made in the mother's abdomen and uterus, and the baby is removed from the uterus. The baby is usually delivered within about the first five minutes of the surgery, and it takes approximately forty-five minutes to complete the procedure. Although a cesarean delivery is considered major abdominal surgery, complications are rare, and with support and pain-relief measures to keep you comfortable, your recovery should go smoothly.

> ### DID YOU KNOW?
> - Approximately 25 percent of all live births in the United States are cesarean deliveries, approximately one million babies per year.
> - Younger mothers have less chance than older mothers of their labor ending up with a cesarean delivery.[1]

The two most common reasons for cesarean delivery are:

1. The mother has chosen to schedule an "elective" cesarean delivery (almost always after a previous cesarean delivery).
2. Labor fails to progress (known as dystocia). Dystocia may be due to a variety of factors. Often it occurs when the baby's head is too big for passage through the birth canal. Dystocia may also be a result of contractions that are not strong enough to move the baby out, or not effective enough to fully dilate the cervix so the baby can pass through.

Other reasons women may have a cesarean delivery are:

• The placenta is blocking the cervix (known as placenta previa).
• The placenta has separated from the uterus prematurely, causing bleeding (known as abruptio placenta).
• The umbilical cord is pushing down through the cervix or vagina ahead of the baby, potentially cutting off the flow of blood and oxygen to the baby (known as prolapsed cord).
• The mother has active genital herpes.
• The baby is in a breech (butt first) or transverse (crosswise) position.
• Either the mother or the baby is in distress (for example, mom spikes a fever or baby's heart rate drops).
• The mother has a medical condition that may indicate the need for a cesarean delivery, such as diabetes or severe hypertension.

WHAT KIND OF PAIN RELIEF IS USED FOR A CESAREAN DELIVERY?

If it is determined that you must have a cesarean due to an unanticipated difficulty during labor, your pain-relief scenario can change dramatically. There are three methods of pain relief used for a cesarean delivery, depending on the circumstances for both mother and baby. If you have been in labor, the most typical form of pain relief used during a cesarean delivery is an epidural. Most scheduled cesareans use a spinal block. Around 10 percent of cesarean deliveries, almost always under emergency circumstances, involve the use of general anesthesia.

EPIDURAL

If you have already been given an epidural during labor, you will simply receive more medicine via the epidural catheter, which will be adequate to provide complete pain relief throughout surgery and recovery.

If an epidural is used, you may receive a dose of a medication called Duramorph, which is morphine. This medication will give you complete pain relief that will last even after the epidural is removed, throughout the hours immediately following your surgery. If you do not already have an epidural in place, typically you will get a spinal block for the cesarean delivery.

SPINAL ANESTHESIA (SPINAL BLOCK)

> Spinals are usually the first choice of anesthetic for women who do not already have an epidural in place.

What It Is and What It Does

The spinal block, also called the spinal, involves injecting a single dose of a numbing medication, with an extremely fine needle, directly into the sac of fluid that contains your nerves and spinal cord. Since the medication goes directly into the fluid around your nerves, it provides almost instant pain relief. Once the medication takes effect you will be completely numb from the chest down.

The spinal is different from the epidural in three distinct ways. First, the medications are administered directly into the spinal fluid (not outside of the sac). Second, the spinal block uses only one injection, and there is no catheter in place to continue to infuse pain-relief medication. Third, the onset of pain relief from the epidural can take some time, often ten to thirty minutes, whereas the spinal block takes effect within a few minutes, usually less than five.

Your Spinal Anesthesia Step by Step: How It Is Done and How It Feels

Step one: While you are curled in a ball-like position on your side or over the edge of the bed, your back will be wiped with a cool antiseptic solution and a paper or plastic drape will be placed over your lower back.

Step two: A numbing medication is quickly injected with a tiny needle into the skin on your back where the spinal needle will be inserted. This may feel like a small pinch, no more intense than what you may feel when receiving numbing medication during a dental visit.

Step three: A thin needle with numbing medication is injected into your lower spine into the sac of fluid containing your nerves and spinal cord. The medication now in your spinal fluid bathes the nerves and spinal cord.

Step four: The anesthesiologist is continuously monitoring your breathing and blood pressure and can help reassure you as you adjust to this altered sensation. The sensation of a numb chest is quite disconcerting to some people. If your hands are not weak and you are

able to talk, you are fine, although you may not feel
fine. Your anesthesiologist will be with you at all times
to help assure you that all is going well during this stage.
One helpful trick for you to employ is to notice the
moisture from the condensation on the oxygen mask
each time you exhale as reassurance to yourself that you
are taking adequate breaths.

Many women report feeling a warm, tingly sensation that
begins in their feet and rides up through their legs and torso as
the spinal medication takes effect. Similar to the epidural, your
legs will feel numb and heavy at first. The medications will take
effect immediately, and very quickly you will feel completely
numb from your toes up to your chest area. Some women report feeling as if they are not breathing adequately. Others feel
a shortness of breath (as if it's difficult to catch a full breath). If
this happens, be assured that it is just the sensation of your
breathing that has changed, due to the numbing effect of the
medication, and that in reality you are breathing just fine.

The numbing medications from the spinal generally last two
to four hours, depending on how much medication is used.
The long-acting pain-relief drug Duramorph is often used in
spinals as well as in epidurals, so when your anesthetic begins to
wear off, you will likely experience only minor (or no) pain for
about eighteen to twenty-four hours. The main advantage of
Duramorph is that since it is put directly into the spinal fluid, it
stays in your spinal cord and provides pain relief to the nerves
without going into your bloodstream, thus making it highly effective in relieving pain, even for the first few hours following
surgery. If you do have some discomfort during this period, additional medications can be given to keep you comfortable.

How *You May Feel When the Spinal Begins to Work*
    How you may feel once the spinal begins to work depends
on what's going on at this point in the birth. If you are having

a scheduled cesarean, you are most likely prepared for the event. You have had time to anticipate the sensations you might experience during this birth and you may be feeling more attuned to the positive feelings of knowing that you are about to meet your new baby in the next few minutes. If you are given a spinal for an emergency cesarean, it is likely you will focus less on the pain-relief measures taking place, and may be more attuned to the shift in activity going on around you, moving from the birthing room to the operating room.

Reason You May Be Given a Spinal

- A spinal is typically used if you are having an elective cesarean. However, some anesthesiologists use an epidural if you are having an elective cesarean.

Medications Used in a Spinal Block

The medications used in a spinal are typically bupivacaine, which is a local anesthetic, a narcotic called fentanyl, and Duramorph, which provides the long-lasting pain relief after surgery.

Your Partner's Role When a Spinal Is Used

Your partner may or may not be in the room when your spinal is given. Most hospitals do not allow the partner to be present during the administration of a spinal, but your partner will most likely be allowed into the operating room during the surgery, to witness the birth of your baby.

Potential Benefits of Having a Spinal

- You will experience rapid and complete pain relief.
- A much smaller dose of medication is used than in the basic epidural.
- The spinal does not cause drowsiness; you can be alert and aware throughout childbirth.

Potential Limitations of Having a Spinal

- Since no catheter is used (as in an epidural), the medications can be given only once. It is only in uncommon situations, when long surgery is a possibility, that more medication may be needed.

Potential Side Effects of a Spinal on the Mother

- Occasional headache after delivery is reported by some women. This occurs sometimes due to leakage of cerebrospinal fluid when the spinal needle punctures the dura. The development of new spinal needles has significantly minimized the chances of your getting a headache as a result of the procedure. Typically, headache occurs about 1 percent of the time after a spinal is given.[2]
- The medications can lower the mother's blood pressure temporarily. This is rarely a serious problem and can be corrected quickly with intravenous fluids or medications, if needed.
- Generalized itching is very common but usually very mild. If you experience severe itching, medication can be given to reduce this side effect.
- Nausea is uncommon but does occur in some women.
- You may have temporary urinary difficulty until the numbness wears off. However, most women have a urinary catheter after a cesarean delivery, so the ability to urinate is not a problem.
- Some women report shivering after receiving a spinal injection. (As noted earlier, this can happen after an epidural, too, and some women who receive no medications during childbirth also report shivering.)
- In extremely rare cases the spinal injection can cause nerve injury or infection.[3]

Potential Side Effects of a Spinal on the Newborn

Only a tiny amount of medication reaches the baby when a spinal block is given.

- If the mom's blood pressure drops, this may cause decreased blood flow to the baby, slowing the baby's heart rate (this is treated right away with fluids and, if necessary, with medications).

Conditions or Situations That May Prevent You from Having a Spinal

- You have a history of blood clotting or take certain medications that can affect blood clotting. You should discuss all of this with your obstetrician or an anesthesiologist prior to going into labor.
- You have certain neurological disorders.
- You have previously had certain lower-back surgical procedures.

GENERAL ANESTHESIA

If there is no time to place an epidural or spinal, general anesthesia may be used to provide instant unconsciousness and allow for immediate surgery.

> General anesthesia is not used to relieve labor pain but is given only in situations where timing is critical, such as an emergency cesarean section or other rare and urgent medical conditions due to the status of the mother or the baby.

What It Is and What It Does

General anesthesia puts you completely to sleep, using medications injected into your vein and gases inhaled via a breathing tube inserted into your lungs after you are asleep. The use of general anesthesia during childbirth is far less common now than even a decade ago. The epidural, the spinal block, and other forms of regional anesthesia, with their safety and effectiveness, have replaced the use of general anesthesia in almost all but the most urgent childbirth situations. Today, general anesthesia during childbirth is used almost exclusively for emergency cesarean deliveries and other rare childbirth complications that require urgent delivery, such as severe bleeding and some types of medical conditions that prevent an epidural from being used (see page 84).

How It Is Done and How It Feels

It takes the anesthesiologist only minutes to administer general anesthesia. If you must be given general anesthesia, you will be completely asleep within seconds. You will remain asleep for the entire surgical procedure, and will awaken in the recovery room. You will not feel pain while under general anesthesia. The effects of general anesthesia may leave you drowsy for a few hours, until the medication wears off.

How You May Feel After General Anesthesia

You may feel relieved that your complicated birth experience or emergency cesarean is now over and the baby has finally arrived. You may also feel disappointed that you could not remain awake and alert to be a part of your childbirth experience. You will most likely not have any awareness or memory of the events that took place while you were under the effects of the anesthesia.

If you have received general anesthesia, it's likely that this was not a part of the plan, and this extreme departure from how you had envisioned giving birth may feel unsettling to you and your partner, even when you have a healthy baby afterward.

After such an experience, you may benefit from talking with your nurse or midwife about how you're feeling emotionally.

Once the general anesthesia wears off, you will likely begin to feel some pain. Often pain-relief medications will be continued through your IV. If you begin to feel uncomfortable, you should let your nurse or physician know.

Medications Used in General Anesthesia

The drugs commonly used for general anesthesia given through an IV are sodium pentothal, propofol, fentanyl, Valium, and midazolam. The commonly used inhalation drugs (gases) are desflurane, sevoflurane, and isoflurane.

What Your Partner Can Do

Most likely, if you are given general anesthesia, your partner will not be allowed to join you in the operating room, since, due to the effects of the anesthesia, you will not be able to interact with him. He will generally be encouraged to join you once you transfer to the recovery room.

Potential Side Effects of General Anesthesia on the Mother

ANNOYING AND UNPLEASANT SIDE EFFECTS

- You may feel drowsy for the first few hours after waking up.
- You may experience dizziness for the first few hours, until the medications begin to wear off.
- You may feel nauseous and experience vomiting throughout the first day after surgery. Medications can be given to ease or eliminate these side effects.
- Your throat may feel sore from the tube that was used to keep your airway open during surgery.

SERIOUS AND RARE SIDE EFFECTS

- The most serious side effect caused by general anesthesia is the possibility of vomiting food or liquid while asleep during surgery, known as aspiration. If some of the stomach contents go into the mother's lungs there is a risk of pneumonia or breathing problems; in extremely rare instances, death may result. By *extremely rare,* we mean: it is estimated that for every ten million births, seven women die due to complications from aspiration.[4] Precautions are taken by the anesthesiologist to reduce the chances of this occurrence. These precautions include: (a) giving an antacid to neutralize stomach acid; (b) after you are asleep, placing a breathing tube down your throat to keep your airway clear; and (c) applying pressure below your Adam's apple to prevent any stomach contents from reaching the lungs before the breathing tube is placed.

  The seriousness of this complication is why the anesthesiologist will always ask how long since your last meal, and this is also why you will be asked to refrain from eating for six to eight hours prior to an elective surgery. If the surgery is an emergency, and you have recently eaten, the anesthesiologist can still administer general anesthesia, but the risk of vomiting and aspiration increases.

- Difficulty inserting the breathing tube is another very serious side effect of general anesthesia. In some cases, this can be a fatal complication. The chance of this complication, known as difficult intubation, increases with pregnancy since often the areas of the mouth, throat, and vocal cords, where the tube must be placed, are more swollen during pregnancy, and enlarged breasts can complicate the procedure, making it harder to properly place the tube. For these reasons regional anesthesia (epidural or spinal) is preferred for operations like cesarean delivery.

Potential Side Effects on the Newborn

The medications used in general anesthesia do cross the placenta, although there is minimal anesthetic effect on the newborn. In fact, very often mothers who are asleep under general anesthesia give birth to babies who are active and awake. Some babies born to mothers who receive general anesthesia do show signs that the medication has entered their system, and they may be sluggish or sleepy at birth. However, mothers who have received general anesthesia have typically experienced some type of emergent condition that required rapid delivery, and this condition, rather than the anesthetic itself, can be the cause of some of the baby's temporary drowsiness.

PAIN RELIEF DURING RECOVERY IN THE HOSPITAL AND AT HOME

Pain relief is not only a vital part of surgery but a very important part of your recovery process as well. Your IV will remain in place for a couple of days after the cesarean section, and you will continue to receive pain-relief medications. Once the IV is removed, your doctor will prescribe oral pain-relief medications to keep you comfortable during the remainder of your hospital stay and throughout recovery.

Women are often sent home with a prescription pain-relief medication to manage their pain after a cesarean. You can reduce your dosage and frequency when you begin to feel better. Some women are comfortable weaning themselves off their pain-relief medication a few days after they return home; others need up to a couple of weeks of pain relief. If you feel you are still in a significant amount of pain when you return home, even with medication, it is best to inform your doctor about your discomfort.

> ### Enjoy Taking Care of Your Baby.
> ### You Don't Have to Feel Pain
> ### After a Cesarean Delivery.
>
> Some women are reluctant to take their medication for fear of becoming too dependent on the pain-relief drugs. You do not need to worry about becoming addicted to the drugs given to you after a cesarean delivery. In fact, if you do not take the pain relievers as prescribed, you run the risk of breakthrough pain: when the pain reliever wears off, pain sets in, and it is difficult to catch up or "get ahead" of the pain, leaving you feeling unnecessarily distressed by pain.

Pain Relief and Breast-Feeding After Cesarean Delivery

Your comfort is important not just for your own well-being but also for your baby's. If you are comfortable after the surgery, then activities such as breast-feeding will be easier. Research has shown that after a cesarean, the short-term use of medications such as acetaminophen, aspirin, and ibuprofen appears to be compatible with breast-feeding. Even narcotics, such as codeine, Percocet, Vicodin, or others can be used while breast-feeding.[5] According to the American Academy of Pediatrics, "Drug exposure to the nursing infant may be minimized by having the mother take the medication just after she has breast-fed the infant or just before the infant is due to have a lengthy sleep period."[6]

COMPLEMENTARY AND ALTERNATIVE PAIN MANAGEMENT AFTER CESAREAN DELIVERY

Many of the complementary and alternative approaches used during labor may also be used during recovery. Women who prefer to use less medication for pain management after a cesarean delivery may continue to use their breathing and relaxation techniques, acupuncture, or self-hypnosis to stay comfortable during their recovery period.

If these nonmedical techniques do not provide adequate pain management after your cesarean delivery, you may want to reconsider the use of pain-relief medications to allow yourself to get comfortable rather than struggling with a painful recovery. Remember, a comfortable mom who is not struggling with pain is better able to focus on the needs of her newborn.

RESOURCES

The Essential C-Section Guide: Pain Control, Healing at Home, Getting Your Body Back—and Everything Else You Need to Know About a Cesarean Birth, by Maureen Connolly and Dana Sullivan (New York: Broadway Books, 2004).
www.csectionguide.com
www.ibreastfeeding.com

Eight

WANT TO AVOID
PAINFUL SUFFERING?
SO DID THEY

*Medical men may oppose for a time the use of anaesthesia dur-
ing childbirth, but they will oppose it in vain; for certainly our
patients themselves will force use of it upon the professions. The
whole question is, even now, one merely of time.*

—James Young Simpson, the first physician
to use anesthesia during childbirth in 1847

PAIN RELIEF DURING CHILDBIRTH:
THE OLDEST OF DESIRES

You are not the first woman in history to seek ways to relieve
pain during childbirth. It is sometimes suggested in childbirth
literature that women's quest for labor-pain relief is a distinctly
modern phenomenon. You have probably heard some variation
on this stated many times: "Women have been giving birth for
centuries without the benefit of modern pain relief." What this
statement does not reveal, however, is that women in almost
every culture have tried to find ways to effectively relieve their

pain during childbirth. Whether we are talking about an ancient herbal tea or a modern epidural, the quest to relieve the pain of childbirth is timeless.

The purpose of this chapter is to give you an appreciation for the fact that at this point in history, you do not stand alone in your desire to experience a comfortable, or even pain-free, labor and birth. Each generation of women before you has sought ways to make their childbirth experience less painful. As you will see in this chapter, some of the methods used over the centuries were innovative, some were quaint, some were hazardous, and some were just plain odd.

In this chapter we discuss the attitudes toward pain relief during childbirth at different points throughout history. This chapter covers:

- Interesting pain-relief methods used prior to the discovery of anesthesia.
- Attitudes toward the introduction of pain relief during childbirth.
- Women's fierce political struggle for the availability of anesthesia during childbirth.
- The pendulum swings back to natural childbirth.
- The modern approach that blends "old" with "new."

INTERESTING PAIN RELIEF METHODS USED PRIOR TO THE DISCOVERY OF ANESTHESIA— INCLUDING THE ODD AND UNUSUAL

The modern era of anesthesia did not begin until October 16, 1846, with the first successful public demonstration of the use of ether for surgical anesthesia at Massachusetts General Hospital in Boston. So, what were women doing to lessen the pain of childbirth prior to this fairly recent medical discovery? There is evidence that methods used to attempt to relieve labor pain were used in the ancient civilizations of Babylon, Egypt, China, and Palestine. Methods based on the use of positive thinking as a means to cope with labor pain included the use of rings, necklaces, and charms thought to have magical powers.[1]

DID YOU KNOW? *Some techniques used to ease labor pain in ancient cultures included inhaling assorted concoctions made of poppy extract and hemp, drinking tea mixtures derived from certain plants, or drinking a beverage sprinkled with powdered sow's dung (sometimes mixed with honey wine).*[2]

Primitive methods based on the use of techniques meant to distract women's attention from labor pain were not significantly different from some of today's pain-relief methods. Some of the techniques used then, such as warm compresses, massage, and herbal teas, are familiar even today.

An early version of warm compress and massage during labor is described by Donald Caton, M.D., an obstetric anesthesiologist and academic historian of obstetric anesthesiology. According to Dr. Caton, "One of the earliest references to the management of childbirth pain appeared in a gynecologic text written in the first century C.E., by a Greek physician. He suggested that the physician 'soothes the pains (by) touching with warm hands and afterwards drench pieces of cloth with warm, sweet olive oil and put them over the abdomen as well as the labia and keep them saturated with the warm oil for some time, and one must also place bladders (containers) filled with warm oil along side.' "

Caton describes the pain-relief potion recommended by a "Puritan Minister well-versed in medicine, by the name of Cotton Mather, who advised women to use potions such as the 'livers and galls of eels, dried slowly in an oven,' or 'Date, Stone, Amber and Cumin seeds' to alleviate their pain."

Mesmeric Pain Relief (Hypnosis)
In 1836—just a decade before anesthesia was introduced for use during childbirth—a French physician and hypnotist, Dr. Gru-

bert, suggested the use of "magnetic sleep" (hypnosis) on laboring women to provide pain relief. The use of hypnosis had already been tried for surgery at this time, but did not gain popularity for use during childbirth. Over a decade later, however, two other successful cases of pain relief through the use of hypnosis were recorded. The American case was reported by Dr. Fahnestock of Lancaster, Pennsylvania, in 1846, only one year prior to the introduction of the use of anesthesia during childbirth.[3]

Bloodletting (Leeches)

In the United States, in the early nineteenth century, bleeding, through the use of leeches applied to the skin, was a widely accepted medical intervention. A statesman and physician named Benjamin Rush recommended using this technique and would bleed a patient through the use of leeches, of up to three or more pints a day. His theory was that the pain of childbirth could stimulate the woman's central nervous system, possibly causing harm, and by bloodletting he could depress the mother's nervous system and avoid any danger caused by labor pain.

The Birthing Stool

For hundreds of years, a short wooden stool, with a hole in the middle (similar to a toilet seat) was used as the most comfortable place to give birth. When the laboring woman was ready, she would squat on the stool to give birth. The birth attendant, by placing her hands under the stool, would then catch the baby.

ATTITUDES TOWARD THE INTRODUCTION OF PAIN RELIEF DURING CHILDBIRTH

Long before the introduction of anesthesia during labor (and for some time after) religion played a key role in determining the experience of childbirth for women. Many religious leaders (almost all of them were men) strongly influenced society's laws and social mores and were opposed to the relief of childbirth pain.

The Scripture was cited as evidence that the relief of labor pain was forbidden, since it describes this pain as a punishment given by God to Eve and her descendants (all women) for having disobeyed him in the Garden of Eden. Religious leaders cited Genesis 3:16: "I will greatly multiply thy sorrow and thy conception; in sorrow thou shalt bring forth children." To avoid the pain of childbirth was to disobey the will of God.

In Germany, in 1521, a physician dressed in women's clothes (men were not allowed to be a part of childbirth during that time) entered the labor room of a woman to attempt to relieve her pain. He was discovered and burned at the stake for his offense.[4]

The belief that the pain of childbirth was a divine punishment prevailed throughout most of history. In fact, opium had been used for centuries by physicians as a pain reliever, and morphine was discovered in the early 1800s, but neither of these pain-relieving substances was given to women during childbirth (in part because physicians were concerned about the risks opium or morphine might pose to both the mother and infant).

In addition to the religious attitudes against the use of pain relief in childbirth throughout history, many physicians felt that the pain associated with childbirth was simply a natural phenomenon that did not require any intervention, including intervention designed to relieve labor pain.

The religious interpretation of labor pain has been challenged in modern times, and most religious leaders (including the pope) do not see pain relief during childbirth as a contradiction to the will of God. In fact, the modern interpretation translates the words in the Scripture used to describe childbirth to mean that women will bring forth children "in toil or labor," meaning hard work, rather than pain.

ANESTHESIA COMES OUT OF THE DARK AGES: A BRIEF TIME LINE

Pain Relief First Used During Childbirth in the 1800s

A SOON-TO-BE-FAMOUS OBSTETRICIAN OFFERS THIS STUFF TO LABORING WOMEN!

In 1846, anesthesia was discovered, and for the first time in history, surgical procedures could be performed without pain. Today we take it for granted, but for thousands of years, surgery and other painful medical interventions took place while the patient was fully aware, conscious, and in agony. The discovery of a substance that could put a patient to sleep while a physician was performing surgery was recognized as an event that would profoundly benefit mankind. This pain-relief discovery was soon applied not just to surgical patients, but also to laboring women.

In 1847, a year after anesthesia was used for surgery, a Scottish obstetrician named James Young Simpson used ether to successfully relieve the pain of childbirth for a woman with a deformed pelvis. He then devoted his career to the advancement of anesthesia used during childbirth, improving the pain-relief substances and techniques of the day and impacting the birth experience of women throughout Europe and America.

THE FIRST WOMEN TO BENEFIT FROM ANESTHESIA: THE ROYAL AND THE WEALTHY

Moral opposition persisted until finally the clergy began to lose its power over the childbirth experience, and in 1853 England's Queen Victoria defiantly chose to use inhalation of chloroform gas to relieve her labor pain during the birth of her eighth child, Prince Leopold. The queen showed her appreciation by bestowing knighthood upon the anesthesiologist who cared for her, John Snow. James Young Simpson, the obstetrician who was making great strides in obstetric pain relief, although not her personal physician, was also knighted by the queen.

Those who were fortunate enough to find a physician willing to provide chloroform soon followed the queen's example. Women who had political and economic power began to challenge the church and medical establishment, demanding pain relief during childbirth in particular, and better maternal and infant care for all women in general.[5]

"I feel proud to be the pioneer to less suffering. . . . This is certainly the greatest blessing of this age and I am glad to have lived at the time of its coming." Fanny Appleton Longfellow, 1847, Cambridge, Massachusetts[6]

The first American woman to use anesthesia during childbirth was Fanny Appleton Longfellow, the wife of the famous poet and scholar, Henry Wadsworth Longfellow. Since anesthesia during childbirth was not yet practiced in the United States, Fanny Longfellow sought out a prominent physician, Nathan Cooley Keep, who was known to be experienced in the use of ether (and who was to become the dean of dentistry at Harvard). In 1847, using a device to inhale ether, Fanny Longfellow gave birth to a little girl, and enthusiastically endorsed the use of this new pain-relieving substance.

Pain Relief Used During Childbirth in the Early 1900s

WOMEN'S POLITICAL STRUGGLE FOR ANESTHESIA DURING CHILDBIRTH

In the United States and Britain shortly after the discovery of anesthesia, the quest for pain relief during childbirth became tied to women's social and political struggles taking place in society. Women's advocacy for the advancement of their own political and economic power included the demand for better health care for themselves and their children.

Improved maternal and child health, and a less painful birth experience, were among the important issues of the time. Medical birth control had not yet been discovered; with almost no control over their reproductive lives, women had many children and spent the better portion of their adulthood pregnant.

Well into the early 1900s childbirth remained dangerous for women throughout the world, even in the more medically advanced Britain and United States. In fact, physicians themselves contributed to the high mortality rate of women and infants by not washing their hands after examining and treating patients. When it was recognized that infections were spread from one patient to another, physicians began the practice of hand washing prior to examining patients. The number of women who died from infection, which was known at the time as childbed fever, markedly decreased.

One of the central issues eventually taken on by women's rights leaders in both the United States and Britain was the availability of a more humane birth experience for all women, not just the wealthy few who had access to physicians and could afford pain relief. During the mid- to late 1800s and well into the early 1900s only wealthy and well-connected women could benefit from the new "miracle" of a pain-free birth, and several organizations sought to remedy this social injustice.

> "One of the most cruel class divisions yet remaining in this country is that rich mothers need not suffer in childbirth as though we were still in the Stone Age, while poorer ones far too often do." From a letter from a British writer that appeared in the publication, *The Lady* in 1942.[7]

The early feminists who championed improved health care for all women and children were frustrated by the sluggishness of the medical establishment to make anesthesia more widely available during childbirth. Physicians in general remained reluctant to offer anesthetics to laboring women for three reasons:

1. Although many patients disagreed, physicians themselves were not convinced that the risks involved to the mother and infant outweighed the benefit of pain relief. Many physicians feared, with good cause, that anesthesia could produce unintended side effects in both mother and newborn.
2. Most births were attended by midwives, not physicians. Midwives were not certified by the government to administer anesthetics.
3. In general, most physicians believed labor pain was a natural part of the process of birth.[8]

This passivity toward women's suffering was met with the creation of several political organizations with the mission of overcoming physician resistance toward the use of anesthesia during childbirth.

THE NATIONAL TWILIGHT SLEEP ASSOCIATION

In the early 1900s, American journalists Marguerite Tracy and Constance Leupp wrote that the success of the campaign undertaken by women urging physicians to rid women of labor pain would "relieve one-half of humanity from its antique burden of suffering which the other half of humanity has never understood."[9]

In 1914 a group of wealthy and politically connected American women formed an organization whose mission was to bring to all women in the United States a new pain-relief technique that had reportedly been used with success in Europe. The twilight sleep method of pain relief combined two powerful drugs, morphine and scopolamine. Morphine dulled the woman's pain, and scopolamine had the unintended side effect of lowering women's inhibitions and producing memory loss.

When given to laboring women, twilight sleep often resulted in women exhibiting bizarre and uncontrolled behavior. Since only a small amount of morphine was used, it was often ineffective against dulling the pain, and it was common for women to thrash about and scream wildly. Unaware of the pain they endured due to the amnesia-producing quality of scopolamine, women often reported a pain-free birth experience.

The women who formed the National Twilight Sleep Association launched a successful campaign for the use of this technique during childbirth. They held rallies and inspired women to demand that twilight sleep be made available for all American women. The campaign was meant to shake the medical establishment into responding to women's pain by providing adequate pain relief to all.

There was one critical obstacle to their well-organized, well-funded efforts: consistently, twilight sleep did not provide adequate pain relief. What it did do (although not always) was erase the memory of women's labor pain. Most women were unaware that due to the loss of inhibition they experienced, physicians often put cotton and oil in patients' ears and blindfolded them to reduce stimuli in an attempt to keep them subdued; in addition, women were often restrained in their beds to prevent them from harming themselves or others.

When one of its most prominent and outspoken advocates died during childbirth, after having received this pain-relief method, the National Twilight Sleep Association came to an end. Although her death was not attributed to the use of twilight sleep, the public had become skeptical of its safety. In spite of this tragic event, which was followed by public expressions of concern about its safety, twilight sleep remained in use in U.S. hospitals until the 1960s.

BRITAIN'S NATIONAL BIRTHDAY TRUST FUND

> "Since chloroform was first administered to Queen Victoria . . . in 1853, normal maternity cases in the wards have had to wait for seventy-six years (and the advocacy of the Prime Minister's wife), to obtain this relief."
> —Virginia Woolf, 1948[10]

In 1928, just a little over a decade after the demise of the Twilight Sleep Association in America, a group of wealthy and politically connected British women formed an organization with the mission to improve all aspects of health care for women and children. During this time in Britain, nearly one in two hundred women died during childbirth each year.[11] The organizers of the National Birthday Trust Fund aimed to reduce this statistic by rallying for improvements in maternity care through funding programs to train professional midwives and maternity nurses, and improving maternity services throughout the country. The fund also supported the creation and distribution of modern pain-relief methods to help the fund organizers reach their goal of making pain relief during childbirth a possibility for all women regardless of their social status or income.

A British physician with financial support from the fund helped devise a small glass capsule that could be broken by the mother or caregiver to release a premeasured amount of chloroform into a face mask, relieving some of the pain of labor, without causing the unconsciousness that often resulted when too much of the substance was given. The production of these capsules was paid for by the fund, which also helped distribute them for free to hospitals serving primarily poor women and families. This endeavor was just one of many undertaken by the fund that promoted its organizers' mission to make pain relief available to all women in Britain.

The 1940s Through the 1970s: Returning to the Past— From Anesthesia Back to Natural Childbirth

Not all physicians or women believed that anesthesia during birth was desirable. Some rejected the use of anesthesia based on their concern over the possible side effects to both mother and infant. Others were concerned about the act of intervention, through the use of painkillers, in the birth process itself. The use of anesthesia during childbirth, the movement of birth from home to the hospital, and the primary role of the physician in the process brought forth a different set of objections from women and physicians.

By the 1950s, birth was now an institutionalized event in the lives of women in the United States and parts of Europe. Women had very little control over their own birth process once the hospital and physician assumed responsibility for their care. This new, institutionalized birth experience was met with opposition by a new generation of mothers and physicians who sought a more natural birth experience, free from all interventions, including the use of pain-relief medications.

GRANTLEY DICK-READ

In Britain, one physician profoundly influenced this shift from advocacy for medical pain relief to advocacy for a natural birth. Grantley Dick-Read, an obstetrician who opposed the use of anesthesia during childbirth, inspired women to believe that "healthy childbirth was never intended by the natural law to be painful." He was one of the first to assert a connection between fear and labor pain. He and other physicians at the time suggested that when women experience fear during labor, it activates a fight-or-flight response, which releases body chemicals that prevent normal functioning of the uterine muscles, causing tension, which then results in pain.

Dr. Dick-Read believed that women should remain free of pain-relief medications, fully conscious and aware to enjoy childbirth. He recognized the importance of keeping baby and mother together shortly after birth and was among the first to encourage fathers to be included in the birth experience.

Dr. Dick-Read was not without his critics, though, then and today. Physicians and others have challenged his conclusion that only fear causes the pain of contractions, and some object to his claim that information and knowledge about childbirth can actually eliminate its pain.

Apart from his detractors, Grantley Dick-Read enjoyed popular support among women who were disheartened by the regimented and institutionalized birth experiences they were having on maternity wards in U.S. and British hospitals. His book on natural childbirth, *Childbirth Without Fear,* published in 1933, is still read today, and his theory on the fear-tension-pain syndrome during birth has inspired the development of other natural childbirth techniques.

ROBERT BRADLEY

An American obstetrician, Robert Bradley, developed a natural childbirth philosophy in the late 1940s that became popular over the next several years. Dr. Bradley believed that women should have a natural, drug-free childbirth experience and developed a birth approach known as Husband-Coached Childbirth. That phrase may sound outdated now, but the inclusion of the husband, not just as a witness to the act of birth but as an active participant in the birth process, was a radically new idea at the time.

Dr. Bradley taught women and their partners to use a particular breathing technique to manage the pain of childbirth. Dr. Bradley believed that with proper education, preparation, and the support of a coach, women could be taught to give birth naturally.

During the mid-1960s, when natural childbirth was becoming more popular and women were embracing new techniques to manage the pain of childbirth, the Bradley method established itself as a popular natural childbirth technique. The Bradley method of birth is still used today in the United States and around the world by women who want an entirely natural childbirth experience.

FERNAND LAMAZE

In the 1940s, an obstetrician from Paris named Fernand Lamaze traveled to Russia where he observed women were using a method called psychoprophylaxis, which involved the use of simple breathing and relaxation techniques for pain management during childbirth. Dr. Lamaze returned to France and developed a number of breathing and relaxation techniques, and promoted the use of labor support during childbirth. Dr. Lamaze advanced the idea that controlled, rapid breathing during labor would divert the brain's attention from the pain caused by contractions and allow women to give birth without medication.

The Lamaze Organization began in the United States in the 1960s and its breathing and relaxation techniques became the most popular birth approach for expectant mothers throughout the country.

The 1980s and 1990s: The Epidural Becomes Popular, Natural Childbirth Is on the Decline, and Women and Their Caregivers Disagree on Birth Options

During the 1980s and 1990s the use of epidurals (regional anesthesia) grew dramatically in popularity. Many women (whose mothers gave birth to them without medication) were now choosing to give birth to their babies using medical pain relief and, in particular, epidurals. The generation of women who fought for a natural childbirth experience had been replaced by a generation of women who once again began to demand a pain-free childbirth. The number of women who received spinals or epidurals during childbirth increased significantly between 1981 and 1997. In large hospitals nationally, the use of epidurals during this time tripled to 66 percent.[12]

Pain Relief in the 2000s: Blending of Both Sides— Medical Pain-Relief Advances and Natural Methods Begin to Return to Labor and Delivery Rooms

In health care in general, over the last decade, traditional medicine has begun to include alternative medicine. More patients and their physicians are opening up to the idea that nonmedical interventions and techniques may be advantageous in maintaining good health. This trend has also impacted the experience of childbirth. More women, even if they request an epidural, are willing to try techniques that even a few years ago were considered outside the mainstream. Techniques and devices that were previously not found in labor and delivery units are now becoming more commonplace. Hypnosis, water immersion, aromatherapy, birth balls, acupuncture, and other nonmedical approaches are now being used by women, often in addition to medical pain relief. The approach to managing the pain of childbirth is moving to more of a middle ground as women and their caregivers recognize the value of including nonmedical pain-relief methods, even as they continue to use epidurals and other medications.

Attitudes toward the use of pain relief during childbirth have changed, and certainly the actual use of pain relief has also changed, with over 80 percent of women receiving some form of medical pain relief during childbirth. However, strong controversy still exists among some caregivers and women themselves concerning the experience of a pain-free childbirth. Even though it has been over 150 years since anesthesia was discovered, the debate over pain-free childbirth continues.

Resources

For history buffs, we highly recommend a book that covers the history of pain relief during childbirth, titled: *What a Blessing She Had Chloroform: The Medical and Social Response to the Pain of Childbirth from 1800 to the Present,* by Donald Caton (New Haven, CT: Yale University Press, 1999).

Nine

DON'T LET THIS
HAPPEN TO YOU

Anesthesiologists, Obstetricians, and
a Midwife Present Birth Stories—Things That Can
Go Wrong with Your Pain-Relief Plans

Even women who have spent over nine months reading books, surfing the Internet, interviewing other moms, and making it a point to be shining stars in their childbirth preparation courses can have a birth experience entirely different from the one they imagined for themselves. Sometimes plans change, and there is simply nothing you or your caregivers could have done differently, and other times unpleasant surprises occur that might have been handled more effectively or avoided altogether.

You may have already discovered, by spending just a few minutes reading birth stories on your favorite pregnancy website, that successful pain management is not always achieved. This can leave some women disappointed or angry. Some women report that their medical pain relief was delayed or not effective. Others tell about how they were committed to using no medications for pain relief, but complications or a prolonged labor resulted in their having to forgo a medication-free childbirth approach. And some women describe their frustration at not receiving the amount of support they felt they needed to successfully give birth free of medical pain relief.

The scenarios in this chapter describe pain-management approaches that reflect very different birth philosophies. From the midwife who describes the birth experience of a woman who had been committed to a medication-free childbirth, who nearly receives an epidural (at her own request), to an anesthesiologist who tells of a first-time mom's complicated and unnecessarily painful childbirth experience for which she was entirely unprepared, the moms and their healthy babies whose birth stories are told here all fared well in the end. You may benefit from the lessons learned according to their caregivers.

In this chapter:

- You will read accounts by childbirth professionals who reveal how pain-management plans can go awry.
- You will see how an unanticipated change can alter your labor experience.
- You will read how to avoid specific situations that can interfere with your ideal pain-management choices.

EVERYONE HAS THE SAME GOAL IN MIND—A HEALTHY BABY

Mark Zakowski, M.D., chief of obstetric anesthesia, Cedars-Sinai Hospital, Los Angeles, California

"I am an obstetric anesthesiologist who has worked in various settings, including both an academic center and a high-volume private practice. I have personally helped more than ten thousand women giving birth.

"This birth story takes place in a well-known private hospital with the largest number of obstetric deliveries in Los Angeles. The labor ward consists of large labor-delivery-recovery rooms where women can labor and have their family and friends visit.

"A first-time mom and dad arrived on the labor and delivery unit in early labor; mom was in her forty-first week of pregnancy. They had attended Lamaze classes and really wanted to go 'natural.' Both are college graduates with careers, one as a finance officer at a bank and the other as a scientist in a biotechnology company. They arrived on the labor and delivery unit with a written birth plan that expressed all the details of how they wanted to experience their labor and postpartum period: She wants to walk around, be connected to the fetal monitor as little as possible, not have an IV, does not want Pitocin, and wants control over her pain medications—preferably no epidural, and no narcotics. They brought with them a birthing ball, aromatherapy oils, and a doula.

"The labor process was slow. After six hours the mom progressed to three centimeters dilation and became increasingly uncomfortable. The obstetric nurse and anesthesiologist explained her pain-relief options. She had been using controlled breathing with each contraction, but was growing tired and needed a rest. She finally accepted an IV and one dose of an IV medication—fentanyl, a short-acting synthetic narcotic. This took the edge off the pain and made her feel better for about an hour. About three hours later, when she was dilated five centimeters, and exhausted, she finally 'gave in' to an epidural. However, the couple was concerned about the baby getting any of the pain medicine, and they did not want any narcotic in the epidural. Mom looked very guilty and apologized for not making it all the way 'natural.' She received the epidural with only local anesthetic and when her pain subsided, she fell asleep, exhausted.

"As she slowly progressed, she needed additional epidural medication. She had a lot of pain on her perineum, or bottom, but she adamantly refused further narcotics in spite of the anesthesiologist's explanation about the safety and effectiveness of epidural narcotics. Thus, only more local anesthetic was administered via the epidural catheter. Her legs got heavy, but she still had some residual pain in her lower back and bottom, so she asked for more pain medicine to take away the lower back discomfort. When it was time to push, her legs were wobbly. She had some difficulty pushing, but did an adequate job. When the baby's heart rate dropped, then recovered, the obstetrician told her, 'We have to deliver you now,' and asked her to push.

"Although she tried hard to push, she couldn't get the baby out fast enough and the obstetrician had to use forceps. The baby delivered 'sunny-side up,' with a cord around the neck. Mom suffered a third-degree tear (a tear of the perineum that includes a partial tear of the anal sphincter muscle). An epidural 'repair dose' was given to allow the obstetrician to sew the perineum."

Dr. Zakowski's Advice:

"Be flexible. Your doctors and nurses will do their best to accommodate your individual wishes. However, respect their suggestions and support. Everyone has the same goal in mind—having a healthy baby. Although the epidural can take away the pain completely for most women, sometimes there are aspects of the labor that will affect how well the epidural works. Remember to work *with* your health care professionals and be flexible on your well-thought-out birthing plan.

"The anesthesiologist accommodated the patient's requests, although doing so made the pain management more difficult. If this mom had accepted the epidural narcotic, the need for local anesthetic would have been reduced, the pain relief would have been better, and pushing would have been more effective. Different situations require different treatment modalities and medications. The anesthesiologist can tailor the medication 'cocktail' you get to suit your individual pain-relief preferences as well as respond to various emergent obstetric situations. Getting an epidural can be of great help not only with pain relief, but also with safety if an emergency arises. The birthing situation can change rapidly, and it is to your advantage to be flexible."

THE BIRTH PLAN—IT'S SUBJECT TO CHANGE

**Ann Rehm, M.D., obstetrician and gynecologist,
William Beaumont Hospital, Royal Oak, Michigan**

"I am a board-certified obstetrician/gynecologist in a northwest Detroit suburb. The hospital where I work is quite large and busy, performing over six thousand deliveries per year. We have a birthing center where patients can labor and deliver in the same room, but go to a separate postpartum wing after delivery. The hospital, however, is a level three center, which means it provides neonatal intensive care and perinatology support for high-risk pregnancies.

"Mrs. Smith came to my practice when she was twenty-two weeks into her pregnancy. She was expecting her first child and came to my office as a transfer of care from another practice. She brought a written birth plan to our first appointment, and stated her intentions for minimal intervention. Mrs. Smith also wanted to have a doula present at her birth.

"At the first office encounter we reviewed her birth plan together as a team. Reasonable requests were agreed upon. Other requests that were more rigid were discussed and annotations were made on the birth plan.

"Mrs. Smith's pregnancy was uncomplicated. At forty-one weeks, she went into labor and arrived on the labor and delivery unit at seven A.M., after laboring at home, with her husband and doula, for seven hours. She was six centimeters dilated with a bulging bag of waters. The baby's heart rate was strong and reassuring. The patient walked and took warm showers. At two forty-five P.M., I examined Mrs. Smith (as per her request to limit cervical checks) and she was still six centimeters. In spite of walking the hallways, rolling on the birth ball, and using the warm shower and aromatherapy, she had not made progress and was agreeable to having her water broken [artificial rupture of the membranes].

"Two hours later, Mrs. Smith began to feel more uncomfortable and felt like she needed to push, but at that point she was only seven centimeters dilated. She took another shower, but was becoming very uncomfortable and feeling exhausted. She desired reexamination, which showed her cervix was still at seven centimeters. At this point, she was distraught and wanted to know if there was anything else 'we' could do.

"I explained that I would like to initiate an IV to rehydrate her [and the baby], to begin Pitocin in an attempt to augment her labor, and to administer an epidural to help her relax. She agreed to go with this plan. She received her epidural and rested in the labor bed. The Pitocin increased the strength and frequency of her contractions, and by nine P.M. she was completely dilated and the baby had descended.

"She pushed for about four hours and made slow but steady progress. She had no desire for a vaginal assisted delivery (forceps or vacuum) and her nap, combined with her sheer determination, seemed to work—the baby began to move down the birth canal on its own. She delivered an eight-pound, twenty-one-inch baby girl without an episiotomy. She had only a small perineal laceration. There was meconium [baby's first bowel movement] visible in the amniotic fluid, so instead of placing the baby on the mom's abdomen, I needed to have the anesthesiologist insert a tube into the baby's throat to see if any meconium had passed into its airway. [The presence of meconium found in the amniotic fluid at birth is a sign that the baby may be in distress.] Thankfully, the baby's airway was clear. The baby still needed to go to the observation nursery for a short time for breathing irregularities, but she joined her parents about three hours later.

"We were all very fortunate to have such a wonderful outcome. The doula helped the patient with massage and breathing techniques without overstepping boundaries, and was not resistant to my suggestions. The patient was happy with a vaginal birth. At the end she asked me why I didn't offer the IV Pitocin and epidural sooner. She said, 'It really did the trick.' I responded, 'It was in your birth plan, "Do not offer analgesia/anesthesia unless requested by mother."' She told me, 'I think I will revise my birth plan for the next time!'"

Dr. Rehm's Advice

"Most likely, if we had broken the bag of waters [amniotomy] earlier and augmented her labor sooner with Pitocin, we may have had a shorter labor course without the complication of meconium in the amniotic fluid. And if so, the baby might have been able to stay in the mother's arms in the delivery room for immediate bonding and nursing. Reflecting back on it now, I think every birth plan should be reviewed by the patient and doctors involved in their care. I believe birth plans should be used as a discussion point. They should be regarded as a tool for ongoing dialogue throughout the prenatal course, as well as throughout labor.

"The patient should realize that we will try to accommodate her wishes, but medical needs will dictate the course of action during labor. Doctors have their patients' best interests in mind when selecting their course of action. The bottom line is: we all want a healthy baby as the final outcome."

YOUR BEST DEFENSE AGAINST DISAPPOINTMENT: REALISTIC EXPECTATIONS, FLEXIBLE PLANS

Gerry Bassell, M.D., obstetric anesthesiologist, Wesley Medical Center, Wichita, Kansas

"The hospital at which I am an obstetric anesthesiologist has a freestanding building dedicated to providing childbirth care to women with routine, low-risk pregnancies. This area is completely separate from the delivery suite in the main hospital and is designed to be family oriented and homelike. Each room is large, with a whirlpool tub, nonhospital furniture, large-screen television, couches and reclining chairs, and an attached but separate room for family members who wish to relax away from the labor environment.

"The mother-to-be requests this birth setting when visiting her obstetrician or midwife during prenatal visits and, as she approaches the end of pregnancy, if she continues to be low risk, she is told that she should go to the low-risk birth center when labor begins. Women who are able to use this setting are encouraged to prepare and bring with them a birth plan to acquaint the nursing staff with their preferences. Sometimes the birth plan is so restrictive and inflexible that the staff's ability to provide safe care to mother and baby is severely limited and a precarious medical situation can develop. Such was the case with Brandi.

"Brandi was a first-time mother-to-be who had originally desired a home birth but was talked out of it by her mother. Her mother was of similar build to Brandi, barely five feet tall, and had been told by her physician, when she was pregnant with Brandi, that she had a very small pelvis. Brandi's mother had experienced a very difficult and painful labor with Brandi before having a cesarean birth. She convinced Brandi that a home birth experience might not be the best choice for a first pregnancy.

"When Brandi arrived at the birthing center in early labor, she presented the staff with her birth plan, which specified, among other things, that she wanted to walk throughout labor until she herself decided to go to bed. She refused continuous electronic fetal monitoring, but agreed to hourly auscultation of the baby's heart [listening to the heart with a stethoscope] by the labor nurse. She did not want an intravenous drip, but if intravenous access were mandated by facility policy, she would accept placement of an intravenous with no fluid attached. She also included in the plan a statement that read as follows: 'I do not want any pain-relieving medication at any time during my labor even if I request it during the later part of labor.'

"When the anesthesiologist on call went to Brandi's room to obtain a medical history and anesthesia evaluation, a routine process that allows early identification of potential problems, Brandi refused to talk to her, saying, 'I won't be needing you or your services.' Despite the anesthesiologist's attempt to explain the importance of obtaining an accurate anesthesia-related history, Brandi's decision was nonnegotiable.

"Brandi continued to walk throughout labor, returning to

her bed hourly to allow the nurse to listen to the baby's heart-beat. At the point where she decided to return to bed for the rest of her labor, examination of her cervix by the nurse revealed that she was three centimeters dilated, with the baby's head not very well descended. Despite the relatively early stage and slow progress of her labor, Brandi was complaining of intense abdominal and back pain. She steadfastly refused all offers of pain-relieving medications, however, when proffered by her nurse. Over the next six hours, Brandi's pain worsened, but her cervical examination revealed only one more centimeter of dilation, without any change in the position of her baby's head. The baby's heartbeat was becoming more difficult for the nurse to locate, so Brandi agreed to continuous electronic monitoring of her baby using an external Doppler technique. The initial tracing appeared normal.

"At this stage, Brandi had been in labor for more than ten hours. Her obstetrician suggested that an intravenous infusion of oxytocin (Pitocin) should be started to enhance her uterine contractions, but Brandi refused. Her obstetrician then broached the subject of possibly needing to perform a cesarean section if the progress of Brandi's labor didn't improve. Brandi wanted to persist with her labor. The nurse informed the anesthesiologist of the possibility of a cesarean section, but once again Brandi refused to talk to her when she visited to ask whether she could obtain an anesthesia history.

"Brandi continued to labor for an additional six hours. Her pain level was increasing and she was becoming physically and mentally exhausted. The baby's heart rate was not as reassuring as it had been earlier, and it was falling with each contraction. Her obstetrician now recommended an urgent cesarean section for obstructed labor with a nonreassuring fetal heart rate, and Brandi consented. She requested an epidural anesthetic so that she could remain awake for the birth of her baby. She was taken to the cesarean section room, where she was greeted by the waiting anesthesiologist, who began to obtain an anesthesia-related medical history that included questions that would not usually be asked by other physicians.

"Brandi's past medical history was normal apart from a complaint of bleeding gums after brushing her teeth. She told the anesthesiologist that this had been occurring since about the middle of her sixth month and happened every time she brushed. It was now too late to check Brandi's blood-clotting ability; the cesarean section needed to be performed relatively quickly. The anesthesiologist explained to Brandi and her mother that she would have to use a general anesthetic for the cesarean section; an epidural anesthetic would not be possible on short notice. The reason for this, she explained, was that an epidural anesthetic should only be used when there is no suggestion of abnormal clotting function. The epidural space is a closed area that could allow pressure buildup against nerves if uncontrolled bleeding were to occur. That sort of bleeding could happen after an epidural if there was any problem with Brandi's ability to form a blood clot.

"Brandi and her mother were very disappointed that she would have to be unconscious during the birth of her baby boy, Randall, and that her mother would be unable to join her during surgery.

"As she was leaving the cesarean section room, Brandi's mother reassured her that everything would turn out well. It did. Randall was born without complications but with a temporarily changed head shape that told the story of Brandi's pelvis being an impossibly tight fit for him."

Dr. Bassell's Advice

"What could have been done differently to avoid Brandi's disappointment and potentially dangerous experience? The literature she read during pregnancy and the prenatal classes she attended should have prepared her for the fact that labor is unpredictable. The duration, the amount of discomfort felt, and the need for additional stimulation of contractions vary among women, and among different labors in the same woman. The key to avoiding disappointment is to maintain flexibility. Making absolute decisions before labor has even commenced can be fraught with problems. Birth plans are a valuable communication tool but must be realistic. Expectations of what will happen during childbirth must be tempered with a healthy dose of realism. Everyone associated with the process of childbirth, from the parents-to-be to the obstetric anesthesiologist, has as his/her primary concern a safe, happy outcome."

Prepare for the "What-Ifs"

Gayle Riedmann, certified nurse-midwife, Oak Park, Illinois

"I have been a certified nurse-midwife for eighteen years, and I am currently supporting women through their labor and birth in a hospital-based alternative birth center. My philosophy as a certified nurse-midwife has been to provide noninterventive alternatives to women seeking a natural childbirth. I describe noninterventive as a birth experience without the use of medical procedures such as IVs, fetal monitors, or medical pain-management approaches. The women who come to my practice are hoping to avoid medicines and anesthetics for labor-pain management. I offer many alternatives to pharmaceuticals and epidurals, including hydrotherapy (water labor and waterbirth), use of massage, birthing balls, squat stools, freedom of movement to change positions (through intermittent fetal monitoring and no IV), and encouraging eating and drinking throughout labor. All of these pain-management options have been demonstrated to assist women through the labor and birth process.

"My discussion with women who interview me about my practice philosophy will include all of the options I have described in the previous paragraph, with one clear theme: 'This is *your* birth. . . . You tell us your hopes and we will help to achieve the birth you want to the best of our ability. But there are no rules here. If you need more pain management during labor, you have to ask; we won't offer. But that doesn't mean you can't ask for more options or our recommendations.'

"Sarah and her husband, Jake, were very well educated

about the birth process. They were both medical health professionals and knew what they wanted. They enrolled in a Bradley
childbirth class to learn the relaxation techniques and alternative options for pain management. This was their first baby, and
they planned to use the hospital's birth center and have a waterbirth. They had some very distinct requests for their birth plan
and hoped to avoid using an epidural or having any pain medicines.

"Two weeks before her due date, Sarah began laboring in
the middle of the night. She called me very excited, delighted
to be having her baby a little early. She and Jake labored at
home for a few hours, using the shower and back massage to
move her through the early phase of labor.

"After only four hours of labor, Sarah called feeling very
uncomfortable with an intense labor pattern. She was caught
off guard by the surge in intensity and felt fearful. We agreed to
meet at the hospital. Although I was uncertain how far her
labor had progressed, I knew she needed the additional support
of her midwife and the birthing room.

"When Sarah arrived at the hospital birth center, she was
moaning loudly with each contraction, verbalizing loudly that
she wasn't sure she could do this. We quickly moved through
the admission process, discovering that she was already seven
centimeters dilated, with a bulging bag of waters. Her husband
and I praised her strength, encouraging her to ride it out, that
her labor was progressing rapidly and she would soon be pushing. Sarah began to feel more frantic, expressing her fears that
she couldn't do it. I reminded her that a fast labor does not necessarily mean an easy labor . . . but that she was already doing
it, and as a matter of fact, was almost done.

"Sarah was not to be consoled. She requested an epidural.
Jake and I reminded her of her goals . . . almost achieved. I reminded her that she was in transition, and that *all* women want
to be done, to escape the process, during transition. I offered
that she try the birthing tub—it was filled and waiting. Water is
excellent pain relief. I asked her to please try it. 'No,' was her
response. Position change also works. I prompted her to try, but

her answer was an unequivocal 'No.' I offered that she could try to give it one hour and by then she would likely be pushing. And I added, if she was not pushing by then, we could move forward with the epidural. 'No,' she said.

"My fear at this point was that by the time the anesthesiologist arrived, and we got the IV started, she would be completely dilated and ready for pushing. I was also concerned that since the epidural can sometimes interfere with pushing by reducing sensation, it might actually prolong her labor. Additional concerns I voiced were that epidurals don't always work, and she would have suffered the difficult task of sitting still for placement while going through transition. I do not feel as if I ever want to talk somebody out of an epidural, but I truly felt that this was perhaps not the best choice for helping her with her pain issue. But my central philosophy always holds true, that it is *her* birth, and while I may have recommendations, the choices are hers. She wanted the epidural.

"We moved Sarah out of the birth center and into a regular hospital labor room, and began the process of starting an IV. It turned out that starting the IV was difficult; after three tries by the nurses, the anesthesiologist was called to start the IV and to place the epidural. He also had difficulty. During this time Sarah was trying to hold still in her bed; fetal monitors were applied, as necessary for an epidural. This whole process was frustrating and agonizing.

"Once the IV was started, I asked Sarah if she would like to be examined for labor progress once more before the epidural was placed. She said yes. Not surprisingly, Sarah was completely dilated. She declined the epidural and began pushing. I took off the fetal monitors and resumed intermittent monitoring, gave her a few swallows of juice, and we prepared for the birth. After twenty-five minutes of pushing, Sarah had a beautiful baby boy in her arms.

"Jake and Sarah were delighted with their rapid labor and short second stage. She did not have an episiotomy and did not have any perineal lacerations. Sarah asked to go back to the birth center room for her recovery and postpartum. Unfortunately, the room had become occupied with another patient, so that was not possible. Sarah was not sorry she had asked for the epidural. She had truly felt she needed it as a rescue from her overwhelming labor contractions. But she did express that she wished she had listened to my words of wisdom at the time. Had she tried only one of my pain-management options, she would have been ready for pushing, and not had to endure the change of rooms and multiple IV attempts. Ah, but hindsight is twenty-twenty, I reassured her. We didn't know that what I had offered would have worked or that she would have been ready to push as fast as she was. But my experience and wisdom told me it was worth a try."

Ms. Riedmann's Advice

"Therein lies the lesson of this birth story. As a woman succumbs to the process of labor, it is overwhelming. That is why we have our husbands or mothers or midwives or doulas to support and advise us. A laboring woman becomes so consumed by the labor process, she is generally vulnerable to suggestions of her support people. In Sarah's case, she did not want to listen to the words of advice or wisdom. She needed to request the epidural to maintain control in her way.

"I was not disappointed for Sarah. Perhaps the demand for the epidural actually helped her cope with her labor. But I would encourage women to listen if they can, particularly if they are in transition, and to try one or two things to help themselves cope before resorting to the ultimate pain-management intervention.

"If you are planning on an epidural or, as in Sarah's case, not planning on one but end up asking for it anyway, there may be glitches along the way, such as the availability of the anesthesiologist, or the effectiveness of the epidural. It is important that you remember your other pain-management coping options and utilize them. Don't 'put all of your eggs in the epidural basket,' because then you are left without a means to cope if something interferes with your plan. Prepare for labor and birth with all options open and considered. Prepare for the 'What-ifs.' "

EDUCATION IS THE KEY

Robyn Faye, M.D., obstetrician, Mercy Suburban Hospital, Norristown, Pennsylvania

"I have been a practicing obstetrician since 1988. In each of the hospitals where I have worked, all small suburban hospitals, my patients have been terrific.

"This birth story involves a very young mother, who successfully avoided learning the basics of childbirth and had absolutely no pain-management plan in place when she arrived at the hospital. Andrea was a seventeen-year-old first-time mom who lived at home with her parents. She had been trying to hide the fact that she was pregnant from her family and friends by wearing her boyfriend's baggy clothes. She told her own parents about her pregnancy on Mother's Day. Her boyfriend left her and her parents were stunned, but planned to help her as best they could.

"Andrea was extremely naïve and immature about the realities of parenthood. She talked about the baby in one breath and her junior prom in the other. Her mom came with Andrea for her prenatal visits, and we talked about her future and expectations. Andrea did not talk; mostly, her mother spoke on her behalf.

"It was clear that Andrea was not confronting the fact that labor would be painful. I tried to get her to focus and to sign up for prenatal classes, but she refused. I talked to her about her options for pain relief, but this seemed to make her uncomfortable. I called Social Services and they agreed that a prenatal class was essential, but she did not attend. I gave her brochures and offered her tapes so that she would not be completely in the dark when she went into labor. I asked her mom to act as Andrea's labor-support person in the labor and delivery unit. I also asked her to educate herself about her daughter's options for pain relief.

"There are five physicians in the practice but I was the physician on call when Andrea's water broke. She had finished school for the day and called to tell me she could not get in touch with her mother. I told her that I would meet her at the hospital and one of my nurses continued to try her mom's cell and office numbers. Eventually her mother was called out of a meeting and arrived at the hospital to greet her hysterical 'child' writhing in pain.

"Getting Andrea back in control was our first job. Her initial exam revealed that she was two centimeters dilated. Andrea was asking for pain relief but was fearful of the IV. She agreed to let us place the IV, and fortunately it was done easily on the first try. The anesthesiologist spoke with Andrea and her mother about an epidural. They chose to go with IV sedation first. I told them that we would monitor her pain and contractions over the next few hours.

"The IV sedation was wonderful. Andrea relaxed well between contractions and was able to get some sleep, but soon she woke up writhing in pain. She was three to four centimeters dilated, and I discussed the epidural. Andrea freaked out at the thought of an injection in her back, but I tried to relieve her fears with my own history of 'three children and three epidurals.' She finally agreed.

"The anesthesiologist arrived and had a very difficult time getting Andrea to stay in position. Finally, the epidural was placed and she was able to relax and progressed to nine centimeters in dilation. Unfortunately, after remaining at nine centimeters for another hour, even with a dose of Pitocin, she did not continue to dilate and needed to have a cesarean section delivery.

"The anesthesiologist added medication to her epidural. Andrea did not seem to understand everything that was going on, and her mom and I tried to explain what was happening. The epidural worked well, and after a stressful and difficult birth, Andrea's baby boy was delivered successfully by cesarean."

Dr. Faye's Advice

"Education is key. Going into labor without knowing what to expect is frightening. Andrea could have used so many different media to get information. There are now many ways to get good information about the birth process and pain-management options—books, classes, tapes, even the Internet. Every hospital offers prenatal classes. Tapes are even available for bed-ridden patients.

"When women know what to expect, I find that they are usually more relaxed. They are still scared and worried, but knowing that the pain will end makes accepting it so much easier. It also makes it easier for the caregivers to help keep the patient focused. No one likes pain, but understanding why it exists and how long it might last enables women to prepare for childbirth and to enjoy one of the most memorable experiences of their lives."

Ten

BIRTH STORIES FROM THE OTHER SIDE OF THE STIRRUPS!

What Happens When Obstetricians, Anesthesiologists, Doulas, and Nurse-Midwives Give Birth?— *Their* Choices for Pain Relief During Childbirth

What happens when the caregiver becomes the patient? Well, the author of the first birth story said it best: "Everything looks different when you're in a hospital gown without your underwear!" In this chapter you will read the personal birth stories from women who have devoted their professional lives to caring for others during childbirth. You will read very different birth scenarios, from the obstetrician who made it clear she wanted no pain, to the doula who had general anesthesia for her first baby, an epidural for her second, then gave birth to her third child, with pain, and peacefully at home. It may be reassuring (and sometimes amusing) to see how the best-informed and the most prepared moms-to-be describe their own birth experiences and their own choices for pain relief.

THE HOLLYWOOD DELIVERY

**Kathryn Zuspan, M.D., obstetric anesthesiologist,
Lakeview Hospital, Stillwater, Minnesota**

"I am an anesthesiologist specializing in obstetric anesthesia. I have been working in academic centers and private hospitals for the last twenty years. I've lectured to hundreds of women in prenatal classes, done countless anesthetics for patients in the labor and delivery unit, counseled thousands of women on pain-relief options, and been present for the sheer joy of childbirth for so many new mothers.

"Was I ready for pregnancy, labor, and delivery? Yes and no. I had a lot of knowledge, which was crucial. Knowing what to expect and all the options that are in your control is very empowering. After years of infertility I finally became pregnant at age thirty-five. I knew that this pregnancy would likely be my only chance at motherhood. I planned to do everything in my power to maximize the health and safety of my little unborn child. I had a lot of book knowledge and experience from my profession. In addition, my father was a well-respected obstetrician specializing in maternal-fetal medicine, so I had an additional excellent resource for all of my obstetric questions. My obstetrician was an outstanding clinician as well as a friend and colleague whom I respected. I would be delivering in the labor and delivery unit where I worked. The labor and delivery nurses were all my friends. My siblings and mother had all had pregnancies and could offer practical tips. I was as prepared for pregnancy as possible.

"How was I unprepared? You can't prepare for the unknowns: all the variances that can occur in pregnancy, labor, and delivery. For example, when I was nineteen weeks pregnant, my cervix started to dilate. I was told I needed to undergo a cervical cerclage procedure. This procedure involves the obstetrician placing a stitch in the cervix, which effectively closes the dilating cervix and prevents potential miscarriage. The procedure required an anesthetic. I chose to have an epidural because I felt that it was the safest option for my unborn child.

The epidural worked well. I was awake and pain-free for the procedure. My baby was exposed to minimal amounts of medication and I went home later that afternoon feeling great. This was my first experience receiving an epidural. I was fascinated by the sensation of numbness. It was similar to the sensation you get in your mouth after the dentist numbs your mouth to repair a filling. I was amazed at how quickly the medication took effect and later wore off.

"I was also unprepared for the sense of vulnerability that goes along with being a patient. Everything looks different when you're in a hospital gown without your underwear. I had heard that it would be weird to experience an epidural because you are essentially letting someone 'stab you in the back.' You can't see what is happening; it is all occurring behind you. When you become a patient you give up a certain amount of control over your life. You suddenly need help or permission to do basic things. I work harder than ever now to help patients maintain as much sense of involvement and control as possible.

"Did I have a labor and delivery pain-control plan? Absolutely. I had a plan that covered labor, normal vaginal delivery, and possible emergency operative delivery. Furthermore, I knew my hospital had anesthesiologists who could carry out my plan. My choice for labor-pain relief was easy. Over the years I had witnessed the results of every possible pain-relief option. I knew which ones worked best. I knew which were safest for the baby and the mother. I didn't need to be convinced that labor was painful. I had heard women screaming, crying, cursing, and threatening their husbands or boyfriends during the throes of labor.

"I wanted an option that would give me excellent pain relief. More important, though, I wanted an option that was safe for my baby. There are a few options that fit that bill, and the epidural was my choice. I knew that I wanted it placed as soon as possible. I knew that I had a great pain tolerance but I also knew that delaying placement was of no value. I didn't want to feel drowsy from any IV medication. I wanted my baby to be awake and alert at birth. I wanted the security of knowing that the epidural catheter was in place in case there was a need for an unexpected surgical intervention.

"This was my labor and delivery plan and it was carried out with great success. Toward the end of my pregnancy I kept two things by my bedside: my obstetrician's phone number and a copy of the anesthesia department's call schedule. I knew that the anesthesiologist was as important as the obstetrician in ensuring the best possible delivery for my baby.

"My cervical cerclage stitch was clipped in my thirty-eighth week of pregnancy. I was surprised when delivery did not follow quickly. Though my cervix slowly opened up to five centimeters over the next several days, I still didn't go into labor. I continued working in the labor and delivery unit, wondering when my turn would come. Finally at seven A.M., on the Thursday morning of my thirty-ninth week, my membranes ruptured (my water broke) as I was dressing for work. I called my husband, Bill, who was making rounds at another hospital (he is also a physician). I also called my parents and in-laws, and made a quick scan of the house to be sure things were decent for company, and then Bill and I headed to the hospital. We were so excited. We couldn't wait to become parents. I still had no labor pains.

"At nine A.M. I was admitted to a labor room, given an intravenous line, and attached to uterine and fetal monitors. My obstetrician said I was seven centimeters dilated. A few small contractions were apparent on the monitor, although I couldn't feel them. The obstetrician's plan was to wait for about an hour to allow for the contractions to improve before considering oxytocin augmentation.

"My plan was to get an epidural before the anesthesiologist who I wanted to do my epidural left the hospital to go on vacation. And he was to leave shortly. So I had the epidural before ever feeling a single contraction. Contractions followed naturally, but thanks to the epidural, I felt no pain with any of them. The most I experienced was a sort of balling-up sensation in my abdomen at the end of each contraction.

"Everyone was pretty jovial. At noon I sent Bill down to the cafeteria with his and my parents. My obstetrician soon said that I was completely dilated and could push if I wanted. I decided to wait until Bill returned from lunch. That is the beauty of a good epidural: I didn't have that frantic 'get-it-out-of-me' kind of sensation that comes at ten centimeters dilation. As I lay pain-free in bed chatting with the nurses, the baby was actually progressing down the birth canal with each contraction. When Bill returned it was time to head for the delivery room, which was used because birthing rooms were not standard at my hospital in 1987. As I passed by the nurses' station on the way to deliver, I smiled and waved. My labor nurse called out: 'This is a Hollywood delivery!'

"In the delivery room I continued to push. I felt no pain, only a pressure sensation. Some women claim they push more efficiently if pain is present. Over the years I've noticed that pain is not a necessary factor. The most effective pushing comes from patients who are not exhausted and who know to bear down with all their might. I pushed with about ten contractions, and our sweet little baby was born at two thirty-eight P.M. She was pink and lively. The obstetrician repaired my episiotomy while we cuddled our daughter. He gave no additional medication and I felt no pain. In fact, the first discomfort I noticed from childbirth was a mild throbbing later that night from the episiotomy repair, but I needed no additional medication.

"The epidural worked extremely well for me, but not all women will have this great an experience even with an epidural. All pregnancies, labors, and deliveries are different. However, I still believe that an epidural can get patients close to the 'Hollywood delivery' and that, frankly, is a great place to be."

FROM GENERAL ANESTHESIA TO AN EPIDURAL TO HOME

Rachel Dolan Wickersham, certified doula

"I've been a certified childbirth educator (first Bradley method, now Lamaze) and a labor-support doula for over ten years. I have worked as a certified nursing assistant to both certified nurse-midwives and direct-entry midwives attending home births, and I work as a doula trainer for Doulas of North America, helping to prepare doulas to work independently. As a doula, I attend to women and their families throughout the birthing process, doing everything I can to empower them by helping them advocate for themselves, and work with their labor, pointing out their strengths and affirming them in their choices. About a quarter of the births I attend as a doula are home births. The rest occur in hospitals across the Chicago area.

"When I became pregnant with my third daughter, I felt fairly prepared. For the birth of my first daughter, I had had an emergency cesarean under general anesthesia. For the birth of my second daughter, I had a successful vaginal birth after cesarean (VBAC). This was accomplished with the aid of Pitocin and, after thirty-two hours of contractions every three minutes, with the aid of an epidural.

"So, with these experiences behind me, I was fairly sure I knew just how intense labor pain could get and, with regard to pain medication, I was fairly sure of what I did *not* want to repeat. My experiences of both the general and the epidural were unpleasant. With general anesthesia, of course, I was 'out' and missed the birth of my daughter. And with the epidural, I felt very uncomfortable with the lack of sensations in my lower limbs and with the feeling that I was unable to breathe. Of course I was breathing, but I could not feel myself doing so. It was quite unnerving.

"In order to maximize my chances of avoiding unnecessary intervention, such as the Pitocin and the use of pain medication, as well as to create the most peaceful atmosphere in which to greet my baby, I chose a home birth. Having done my research, I knew that a planned, midwife-attended home birth was a safe option. Having attended several home births by then, I could also see the advantages of such a choice. I made sure I had good support, inviting my sister and a close friend to attend as my doulas, and I went about planning my home birth. My professional experience as both a teacher and doula bolstered my confidence that with good support and in a space that felt safe and familiar, my home, I could handle the pain.

"Based on my prior birth memories, I knew it would hurt, but I did not fear it as much as I feared repeating my medicated experiences. I was not unrealistic, however, and did all I could to prepare for the expected pain. I had hot packs and cold packs ready, a birth ball, massagers, and aromatherapy all available for use. These items were all pulled out of my own doula bag that I carry when I go to births. I asked my husband, Jim, a wood-worker, to make a birth stool for me so I could sit comfortably to push, and he did. I also asked him to install a full-sized Jacuzzi for me to labor in, and he did that, too. (We happened to be re-modeling our bathroom, so it was not as tall an order as it might seem.)

"When I went into labor, I was somewhat fatigued. My bag of waters had been ruptured for some time and I was feeling a need to get labor going. After spending a long day fruitlessly walking miles with my husband, I had taken a nap and then, with my midwife's approval, gotten up at four A.M. to take some castor oil. It definitely worked, but it left me dealing with some particularly nasty cramps at the onset of labor. I was therefore not in the best frame of mind. However, as the in-tense cramps calmed down and the more normal rhythmic menstrual-like cramping of labor picked up, I became more ex-cited. I woke my husband and called my midwife. The contrac-tions remained five to ten minutes apart for a few hours, never getting very painful, and then gradually began spreading out and getting easier. I felt frustrated because they were clearly not 'painful enough' to produce a baby. Sure enough, by the time my midwife arrived, labor had all but disappeared. She stayed anyway. I watched her unpack her bag and went right into rip-roaring active labor. As so many of us birth professionals know, it was all about emotional comfort. I needed to know she was there. Once I knew that, I could let go and get on with my labor. My earlier contractions had been far apart and gentle, but these were now very close together, about three minutes apart, and very strong. With each contraction I felt carried, as if on a powerful wave.

"Remembering my own work as a doula, I kept myself well hydrated and consciously kept myself upright and leaning forward holding on to someone, or with my hands planted on a surface. I allowed my belly to dangle loosely and I relaxed as many muscle groups as possible in order to allow my body to do its work with as little interference from me as possible.

"I rocked in rhythm with my deep breaths. I also found my voice and allowed my birthsong, the beautiful, deep tones that many birthing women make, to come out. More than anything, the expression of those tones gave me incredible pain relief. Had I been in a clinical setting and felt inhibited, I would not have fully vocalized and therefore would not have been able to handle the pain. But at home I felt free to do whatever I needed to do, including vocalization, to get through the pain. And interestingly, although I definitely felt that each contraction was very, very powerful, I did not feel that any of them were 'painful enough' to produce a baby.

"Yet before I knew it, within an hour and a half of starting my active labor, I felt a sudden urge to push. Labor was over and the hot packs and cold packs, massagers, and aromatherapy all still stood on the dresser unused. I had not even ventured into the bath. All I had left to do was push and I'd have a baby in my arms. Labor had been more than doable. It had been downright simple. Suddenly, however, things changed and this is where I experienced pain for which I was totally unprepared.

"For whatever reason, this little daughter of mine did not descend through my pelvis in the usual manner and she became somewhat stuck. Pushing had been no problem for me the prior time, so I had not given it so much as a moment's thought. Now here I was pushing as hard as I could and not budging my baby at all. And to push and have a baby go nowhere is the most painful thing I've ever experienced. I had not anticipated this.

"Suddenly, my confidence was gone. I panicked and pushed and panicked and pushed and therefore would not have pushed very effectively even if I could have. I kept changing positions, casting about for something, anything, that felt good, but nothing did. My midwife and doulas, confident that I could do it, offered gentle suggestions. I tried them all, but as time passed and the pain became almost unbearable, I became scared. What if I couldn't get her out? How could I possibly transport to the hospital in a car when in this much pain? I clung to my husband, refusing to let him go. I wailed and I prayed. Something needed to change.

"During a strong contraction, I turned my body abruptly as if rolling from side to side and suddenly something clicked, almost as if I'd had my spine chiropractically adjusted, and my daughter came all the way down the birth passage in one push. The feeling of her descending through my pelvis was a bit unnerving. It really helped me relax just by having my midwife and doula affirm me by stating, 'Yes, it does feel strange, doesn't it? But you know all these feelings are normal.' And when I relaxed, it was all manageable. Crowning [when the top of the baby's head exits the vagina] was intense, but I felt prepared for it. Pain gave way to numbness as it usually does, as my baby filled the space. I pushed once more and her head emerged and then she got stuck again. This time my wonderfully skilled midwife went in after her, rotating her shoulders so she could become unstuck. This felt strange, but not particularly painful as I was already experiencing the natural numbing brought on by my baby filling the space so tightly.

"Suddenly, our daughter emerged, none the worse for her brief dystocia. She was lifted up into my arms, where she was greeted joyfully, massaged, and after a time, breast-fed. She never left my arms except to say hello to her daddy after about an hour of nursing. All procedures were done in my arms or on the bed as I sat on it with her. I was so happy, and she was so present and alert the whole time that I forgot entirely about my labor pain.

"In the end I pretty much got what I expected. As I'd seen with my clients, labor was something I could do, and labor pain was something I could manage, as long as I was in the right setting and had lots of good support. Yes, there was a particularly hard part of labor and yes, that part was a big surprise, but even when a woman reaches a point during labor when she believes she cannot go on, she does go on, and with good support, one way or another, she gives birth.

"Remember that much of giving birth is about feeling emotionally safe. Find the place and caregiver with which your heart, not your intellectual brain, feels safest. Choose good emotional support, a doula to help your partner help you, and do everything you can to keep your body healthy and in shape for the birth."

AN INDUCTION, AN EPIDURAL, A BABY

Suzan Ulrich, Dr.P.H., certified nurse-midwife, chair of midwifery and women's health, Frontier School of Midwifery and Family Nursing

"Having your first baby at age forty is exciting. Especially if you are a midwife. At the time of my pregnancy, I was the director of a birth center on the north shore of Boston, where I had been a student midwife thirteen years before, and had learned the art of midwifery from three fabulous midwives, Joan, Fran, and Debbie, who were all still working there. I knew, when it was time, that these midwife mentors would enable me to give birth to my long-awaited little one.

"I kept my pregnancy a secret from the midwives until we had our holiday party. When I disclosed that my 'Christmas wish' had come true, the midwives were stunned and happy. Besides the joy for my news, there were other reactions. Dr. E., the medical director of the birth center, responded that she would 'get the knife ready' for my delivery. She expected that at age forty, at four foot eleven and overweight, I was destined to have a cesarean section. I know the midwives were concerned about me and wanted to make sure all would be well.

"I had no illusions about my pregnancy and birth, no dreams of the perfect birth. I was forty years old and my only desire was for a healthy baby. I wanted to have a natural birth at the birth center where I had attended so many other women and their families during labor and birth.

"For pain relief during labor, I wanted to use position changes and the tub, if all went well. I knew that my mother, who was built exactly like I am, had given birth to me with my arm over my head, and to my brother, who was breech. So, I thought as long as I did not have a big baby, I would have a vaginal birth. But more important to me was a healthy baby, and if that meant a hospital birth, or even a cesarean section, that was fine. I would not feel disappointed.

"Three weeks before my due date, on a Saturday evening, I was trying to rest. I noticed some fluid that was pink tinged. I was sure my bag of water had broken. I felt excited. It was just a trickle, not a big gush. I waited for contractions, but all I felt was a backache. I slept on and off that night and woke at dawn. I knew it was time to see the midwife on call to determine if my water really was broken. I felt an urgency now since nothing had happened all night.

"My husband and I hurried to the birth center and the midwife confirmed my water had broken. After talking with Dr. E., it was decided I would go to the hospital for an induction of labor. I was a bit concerned about this, but knew the midwives, physicians, and nurses would take good care of me.

"I was given Pitocin to stimulate my uterus to contract and to begin my labor. It started slowly and took a while for me to begin to feel much. Dr. E. decided she would examine my cervix. This proved to be way more than an examination. She not only checked my cervix; she stretched it. The feeling was one of intense tearing inside me and I just about jumped up to the ceiling. This stretching sure changed everything fast. Now I was getting contractions that started at the peak with no gradual buildup and release, as with natural labor. The Pitocin caused the contractions to come on like a steamroller. They started at their highest intensity and stayed like that, ending abruptly only to strike again.

"Things were moving fast and the pain was intense. I was sitting up on the edge of the bed almost jumping off to get away from the labor pains. I said to the midwife, 'I am going to die.' She looked directly into my eyes, holding my gaze, and calmly said, 'Don't say that.' She knew the power of words and wanted to pull me back from the brink of fear. I realized she was right. I said, 'No, I know I am not going to die.' But I decided I needed an epidural.

"While waiting for the epidural I begged them to turn the Pitocin down, or off, since I knew it was the medicine in the machine that was making this pain so intense. I am not sure the nurses wanted to do this but the dear young midwife who had done her internship at the birth center, and who was now on staff, turned it down. I just felt I needed a chance to catch my breath so I could get ahead of these contractions because there was no preparation or gradual buildup of the pain. Each contraction hit like a punch.

"I was helped into the shower to let the warm water soothe me. At first the water felt scalding hot on my back, but when it began to feel better, I could focus again. The contractions had spread out a bit, giving me a chance to collect myself while I waited for the anesthesiologist. He finally arrived and gave me my epidural. It was wonderful having the pain go away. But I cried out to everyone in the room, 'I can never be a midwife again. How can I help women in labor anymore since I had an epidural?' I repeated this over and over as everyone in the room laughed.

"I settled down. The Pitocin was increased and labor progressed. In a few hours, it was time to push. As I was pushing, Dr. E. and my midwife, Joan, were at the foot of the bed watching as my mom held one leg and my husband held the other. I stopped in the middle of a push and asked them, 'Is it really going to come out?' I had reached that juncture all women reach where they cannot fathom that this miracle of birth is possible. They said in unison, 'Yes, it will.' I was astonished, but got down to business and pushed. Joan worked her magic using her hands and oil to stretch my perineum so that my little one slid out into her hands. There was my baby. She latched on and nursed well.

"I was very happy and pleased with myself because I had given birth vaginally and had not needed a cesarean delivery. I even felt content about needing the epidural. I had not planned on having an epidural, but I also never planned to have an induction of labor. So I did what I needed to do to complete my journey through labor and come into motherhood."

I'LL WAIT AND SEE

Cynthia A. Wong, M.D., director of obstetric anesthesiology, Northwestern University, Feinberg School of Medicine, Chicago, Illinois

"I have had four childbirth experiences, two actual ones [birth children] and two virtual ones [adopted children], and although they were each unique, they were all influenced by the fact that I am an anesthesiologist who spends a lot of time in a large maternity hospital, taking care of women during childbirth, often administering epidural pain relief for labor and anesthesia for cesarean deliveries.

"I admit to a bias that epidural pain relief is the way to go. I had heard hundreds of women say, 'I did not think the pain was going to be this bad,' and 'I thought I could handle it,' or 'How do women ever give birth without an epidural?' Therefore, I thought that in all likelihood I was going to ask for epidural pain relief for labor, but like many women, I also thought to myself, 'Maybe it is not as bad as everyone says it is and I won't need the epidural. I'll wait and see.'

"I attended an abbreviated Lamaze class for people who had already taken the class and for those with professional childbirth experience. I have to admit that I did not think I was going to be using the breathing techniques that were taught. But it was good for my husband [a nonmedical professional] to attend class. I think I was less worried than most women about labor pain. I knew what to expect and how to fix it. Also, before my first pregnancy I was the regular victim of severe menstrual cramps, especially in the days before Motrin and Advil came on the market, and I imagined this is what labor would feel like.

"I waited anxiously as my due date came and went. I

worked up to the end. I spent the day before going into labor in the cardiac operating room, anesthetizing several patients for open-heart operations as I listened to the cardiac surgeon make jokes about my rotund body habitus. I went to bed early and was awakened suddenly several hours later by a huge 'pop' in my belly. Immediately afterward I had a very painful contraction as fluid came gushing out (luckily I had anticipated my membranes rupturing while in bed and was sleeping on a towel). The contractions continued to come. I was surprised at how painful they were right from the beginning; there was no ramp-up. I woke up my husband and called my obstetrician, who told me to take a shower and come to the hospital. Taking a shower was a good idea. Somehow one feels better when clean, even when having painful contractions.

"The pain was bad but manageable, mostly because there was a break in between contractions. Unlike my menstrual cramps, which continued unabated for several hours, this was a little better. I was examined once I arrived at the hospital. My cervix was dilated three to four centimeters. I did not see any reason to continue to experience the painful contractions. The request for an epidural was not a hard decision for me. I knew I probably had another eight or more hours of labor ahead of me and I saw no reason to continue to experience pain when a safe alternative existed. I never really considered other methods of pain control. I did, however, use some breathing techniques until the epidural medication started to work and I found them useful.

"At some point an intravenous oxytocin infusion was started in order to keep my labor moving along. Long labors after the membranes are ruptured increase the risk of infection. The most anxious part of my labor came when the baby's heart rate suddenly decreased. I automatically flipped around in bed, thinking that the baby was lying on its umbilical cord. I was really having a long contraction (which I did not feel because of the epidural) and this was decreasing the blood and oxygen flow to the baby. I was given a medication to relax my uterus and the baby's heart rate increased to normal, but this had the unfortunate side effect of stopping all my contractions, and therefore my labor.

"In general, I am not an anxious person. I think this is one reason I am a good anesthesiologist: I do not lose my cool when the unexpected occurs. Still, at this point I was anxious to deliver my baby. The contractions became more painful as labor kicked in again. A colleague gave me more medication through my epidural catheter. Now it was time to push and I felt too numb and weak. I really wanted to push so I could deliver, but I felt like I was not being very effective. Eventually I became less weak, and after several hours of pushing, my oldest daughter was born, virtually hairless, but otherwise beautiful.

"My husband was very helpful throughout (except when he announced after the head was delivered that it was a boy), but I think that was because he was well trained (by me) in what to expect. My professional experience is that support people are often very helpful, but sometimes, when they project their own anxieties onto the mother, they can make the mother more fearful.

"An anesthesiologist does not interact with many women after delivery so I was less prepared for the postpartum period. It was more uncomfortable than I had anticipated and I remember thinking that no one had warned me that the effects of pregnancy and childbirth do not disappear instantaneously after childbirth. I was given ice packs for my painful and swollen perineum, and ibuprofen (Motrin or Advil) helped both this pain and the crampy pain caused by the uterus shrinking back to size.

"My second actual childbirth was a slightly different experience. I had slipped a disc in my lower back when I was two months pregnant. A piece of the disc was sitting on one of the nerves to my leg. This caused excruciating pain, much worse than my labor pain. I could barely move for several weeks.

"Going into labor the second time I was not at all anxious about labor pain, but I was scared that I would injure my back again. My second labor started more gradually than my first. I awoke in the middle of the night with contractions that were mild and well spaced out. Recognizing early labor, I attempted to relax and not wake anyone up. Gradually my contractions became more frequent and painful and I got up and took a shower. I woke up my husband and called the neighbor to watch the kids. By the time I arrived at the hospital about four hours later, I was ready for pain relief.

"My second epidural experience was slightly different from my first. This time I received combined spinal-epidural pain relief. The major difference was that a less-concentrated anesthetic solution was used to maintain pain relief, meaning that I was much less numb and weak. However, there was one spot low on my abdomen that perversely hurt no matter what the anesthesiologist did to try to alleviate it. Still I liked this technique better than the first epidural. I was better able to push when the time came (although second babies usually come out more smoothly than first-timers anyway). This daughter's heart rate also abruptly decreased during pushing and my obstetrician elected to apply forceps to her head to help me deliver her more quickly. This did not hurt—one of the perks of epidural pain relief.

"Would I have done anything differently given the chance? No. Do I have some advice? Yes, I do. Women should get educated about pain-management options available during labor. They should help educate their husbands or support people. They should make a preliminary plan, but be ready to change it as the situation demands. And they should not feel guilty about changing it."

THE BEST-LAID PLANS CAN STILL GO WRONG, EVEN WHEN YOU KNOW PEOPLE

Lauren Streicher, M.D., obstetrician/gynecologist and author of *The Essential Guide to Hysterectomy*

"I am an obstetrician/gynecologist in Chicago. I started delivering babies in 1981, and roughly forty-five hundred babies later, my last baby in July 2004. I retired early from obstetrics because of the medical malpractice crisis in Illinois, which I feel has made it virtually impossible for obstetricians to continue to afford to deliver babies. I am currently a health care journalist and write a regular women's health column for a large Chicago newspaper.

"As an obstetrician, I felt extremely prepared for the labor experience, including the expectation that at any time the unexpected could happen. Like most obstetricians, my perspective was a little different. I had no concern about anything as 'trivial' as the need for an IV, an episiotomy, or perhaps a cesarean delivery. My fears were more along the lines of fatal, near-death experiences, but apart from that, I was feeling quite in charge.

"I had a very specific pain-management plan. I wanted the ultimate 'princess' delivery. No pain if at all possible. I felt very strongly that I wouldn't ask a woman to have surgery without pain medication. Why should a women have to endure unnecessary pain on what should be the happiest day of her life? I knew I didn't need to feel pain to love my baby. One of my close anesthesiologist friends had agreed to come to the hospital and place my epidural the minute I had the slightest inkling that I might be in labor. I did try to negotiate to have my epidural catheter placed *before* the onset of labor, but there was only so far my friend was willing to go.

"But, as they say, the best-laid plans . . .

"My bag of water broke at two in the morning, three weeks before my due date. The night before I had been up all night delivering a very premature baby that ultimately died a few hours after birth. Needless to say, I was emotionally and physically exhausted and desperately needed to get some rest. I knew my bag was broken, but since I wasn't feeling any contractions, I opted to just pretend it wasn't really happening and turned over to get a few hours of sleep. At six A.M. I got up and told my husband that we needed to get to the hospital and get my labor going since my bag was broken. Unfortunately, my husband was in the throes of pneumonia and was sick as a dog. Even though he felt far worse than I did, he assumed the traditional father-to-be role, and insisted on driving to the hospital.

Once we arrived I tucked him into a cot in the labor and delivery suite and encouraged him to get a little more rest.

"I suddenly remembered that my obstetrician, Dr. W., had undergone a hysterectomy three days earlier. She had timed her own surgery, anticipating that she would be fully recovered by the time I went into labor. Worse, my anesthesiologist friend was skiing in Colorado. No one had anticipated that my first baby would be three weeks early and I faced the reality that I had a broken bag, no obstetrician, and (gasp!) *no anesthesiologist*. My first and most immediate goal, therefore, was to find an anesthesiologist and get my epidural placed before I experienced an actual contraction. As I started to mull who I would call, the first contraction hit. A way-too-cheerful nurse encouraged me to breathe through it. I informed her that I had no intention of breathing through anything and that she could make herself really useful by finding out who from anesthesia was available. Fortunately, another anesthetist friend of mine heard I was there, arrived on the scene, and placed my epidural. Happily numb, I began to contemplate who would deliver my baby. Moments later I looked up and saw Dr. W. walk into my room (in her hospital gown) saying, 'Let's get this thing going.' Through the hospital grapevine she heard that I was in the labor and delivery unit. She insisted that she was feeling well enough to deliver my baby even though she was still a patient herself recovering from major surgery. It was like a bad movie. My husband in a near coma, gasping for air, my obstetrician in a hospital gown bent over, and a way-too-cheerful oblivious nurse. I was clearly the healthiest one in the room. Nevertheless, the Pitocin got started, I started to have real contractions, and I made very fast progress. I felt virtually no pain other than a little pressure. I rested, read, and chatted with colleagues who stopped by to wish me well and visit my obstetrician (the *real* patient), who sat in the rocking chair by my side. Her husband came with flowers (for her) and ended up giving them to me. My husband slept the day away.

"By one in the afternoon, I was ready to push. We all got

into position. My husband forced himself to get up to "coach" me, my obstetrician took her place at the end of my bed, and her partner stood behind her in case she should faint or not be able to continue the delivery. As I started to push (numb to the armpits . . . just what I wanted), my highly trained ear picked up a drop in the baby's heartbeat. I immediately said to the nurse, 'Get the forceps!' My obstetrician said, 'Shut up and push!' So I did. And in a matter of minutes a tuft of dark hair was followed by my beautiful Rachel Shaina Zar, screaming and full of life. The baby who arrived three weeks early with no obstetrician, no anesthesiologist, a sick father, and an exhausted mother entered the world healthy and ready to take on whatever challenge might present itself."

I WAS NOT AFRAID OF THE PAIN, JUST CURIOUS

Medge D. Owen, M.D., anesthesiologist, associate professor of obstetric anesthesiology, Wake Forest University, Winston-Salem, North Carolina

"I was no stranger to the land of labor and delivery when I gave birth in 2002 at age forty. In 1989 I entered the field of obstetrics and gynecology. I loved to deliver babies but as a young resident doctor, I saw numerous obstetricians burn out by the long hours and worsening malpractice climate. So, after a year of OB/GYN training, I redirected my career to anesthesiology with the intention of becoming an obstetric anesthesiologist. Now, more than ten years later, I still find obstetric anesthesia gratifying; I experience the miracle of childbirth on a daily basis, I help make a painful and frightening experience enjoyable, and I share with parents the joy of one of life's most sacred moments.

"I delayed pregnancy until I established my career but soon learned that becoming pregnant at age thirty-eight wasn't easy. Two miscarriages later, I became pregnant again at thirty-nine. I was understandably a bit anxious when I went for my first ultrasound on September 11, 2001. Indeed, it was a day of shocking events. At the moment I learned the Twin Towers in New York City were under siege, I also learned I had twins in my womb. Two weeks later, one of the fetuses died. The news brought more mixed emotions. On one hand, I grieved another loss, but on the other, I knew that with a single gestation, complications and prematurity would be minimized.

"My pregnancy was uneventful. I was nausea-free and blessed with productive energy. In addition to my normal workload, I organized a woman's fund-raising luncheon for a U.S. senator and started a nonprofit organization to promote safe childbirth in developing countries. As the delivery day drew nearer, however, I became anxious.

"The birthing process seemed less frightening to me than the idea of actual motherhood. I took comfort in the fact that I had seen practically every obstetric complication known to womankind. I also knew how swiftly and gracefully my nursing and physician colleagues handled emergencies, even life-threatening ones, with good outcomes. I had great trust in my health care facility and knew that I would be well cared for. Although I do recommend them, I did not take the childbirth preparation classes, because the breathing exercises were already familiar to me.

"In the late stages of pregnancy, it was fun administering epidurals to patients over my own pregnant belly, knowing that in days I could be on the receiving end. Those same days were bittersweet, because I couldn't conceal my pregnancy while administering anesthesia to women suffering miscarriage. At least I could relate to their sadness, having experienced my own pregnancy losses.

"I scheduled my birth by induction at thirty-nine gestational weeks, and on that day, after a quick shower and coffee (for everyone else), we arrived at the hospital at seven-thirty A.M. It felt strange walking into my workplace knowing that I would be on the 'other side' that day. But the feeling vanished when my boss (typical male) spotted me in the hallway and asked if I could help 'find a lost beeper' before I got started!

"The first three and a half hours of labor weren't bad at all. I could see that I was having regular contractions on the monitor but they weren't painful. By late morning the contractions were stronger. I would pause from my conversation for focused breathing during contractions, which felt like heavy menstrual cramps. My cervix was rechecked and I was two to three centimeters dilated. By noon, my contractions became progressively stronger. It was a type of deep searing and cramping pain, almost indescribable.

"I closed my eyes and went somewhere within myself for about an hour. I created a visual mental image, and with each contraction I pictured myself standing on a white sandy beach with warm, crystal-clear water lapping over my feet. I don't know where the image came from, but it helped me focus, breathe, and remain in control. During this time, a nurse friend came in and set up a CD player with some lullaby music. It was soothing and incredibly helpful for focusing.

"Throughout my pregnancy and up until that moment, I hadn't decided for or against an epidural. If I needed one, I would get it. It was as simple as that. From a medical perspective, I was eager to feel and experience the pain of labor. I wasn't afraid of it, just curious. I preferred not to have a narcotic or other intravenous medicine because I wanted a clear mind. But after over two hours of strong contractions, I knew I didn't want to do this for several more hours. I wanted the epidural and I called for my colleague. I preferred having a CSE (combined spinal-epidural) and we briefly discussed the medication doses. The events seemed surreal and in slow motion as I sat up on the side of the bed and asked my husband to stand in front of me to steady my shoulders. My colleague cleaned my back with antiseptic solution and applied the sterile drape. The numbing medicine was injected under my skin. There was a pressure sensation but it didn't really hurt. As my colleague guided the epidural needle, my father, also an anesthesiologist, and my husband, who is also a physician, were standing over him while he worked. Yikes! I felt pressure in my back more to the left side as the needle was advanced. I informed my colleague of this and he straightened it out. The epidural was placed and as I lay back down in the bed, my water broke. Within three minutes, a warm wave of relief came over my body. The labor nurse checked me and I was five centimeters dilated. I took a deep breath and suddenly realized I was pain-free. Everything relaxed. It was liberating. I saw that I was still having contractions, yet I was comfortable and could freely move my legs. It was a textbook-perfect anesthetic.

"I had no pain. About three hours later, I felt a slight amount of pelvic pressure. My nurse checked me and I was fully dilated. My obstetrician came in and wanted to delay pushing for one hour to let the head naturally descend into the birth canal. An hour later, I put my legs in the stirrups to pre-pare for pushing. My nurse coached me through one push and it went well. I could feel my baby's head in the birth canal. There was pressure and fullness, but no pain. By the third push, I could tell I was making rapid progress. My doctor barely had time to put her gloves on. On the fourth push, my body was expelling my baby through the birth canal even though I was trying not to push. I felt her come out with a big gush of liq-uid. When I saw her, I couldn't believe my eyes. She was the most beautiful baby I had ever seen. She was petite, with a round head, dark hair, and the sweetest cry. It was delightful. I held her on my tummy, dried her, and checked her breathing. The room of family and friends erupted in emotion. Everyone was crying and taking pictures. It was a magical moment.

"Following delivery, I took Advil for pain. I had a burst of energy and intense hunger. Breast-feeding was initially frustrat-ing and painful but I stuck with it. For two weeks, I could feel that spot in my back where the epidural had been placed, espe-cially if I moved a certain way or had clothing rub against it. It was a peculiar sensation, difficult to describe, but only mildly painful.

"The experience of childbirth exceeded my expectations. My years working in labor and delivery prepared me well men-tally, but nothing could have prepared me for the raw emotion and exhilaration. One just has to experience it. The pain was more intense than I expected, but only for a short time. I'm glad I felt the pain and I'm glad I had the epidural. It worked better than I expected and, having had one, I can better coach my labor patients in what it will feel like. The day my daughter was born was one of the best days of my life. If asked one word to describe the experience, it would be 'fun' (and no, I'm not crazy). It was fun because it was filled with excitement, because there was uncertainty about exactly how things would go, and because my family and friends were with me to share the experience."

Eleven

HOW YOUR CAREGIVER'S ATTITUDES CAN IMPACT YOUR CHILDBIRTH EXPERIENCE

Perspectives from the Front Lines—Obstetricians, Anesthesiologists, Labor and Delivery Nurses, Doulas, and Midwives *Tell It Like It Is*

Pain relief is not the only factor that contributes to your sense of satisfaction during childbirth. The amount of control you have during childbirth, whether your expectations are met (or not), and the role of the caregiver are all contributing factors that influence your sense of satisfaction with your overall childbirth experience.

A positive birth environment provides a birth experience in which you will feel safe, well cared for, listened to, and supported by those around you, including your partner and/or family members. The factors that will (or will not) allow this to happen include "the attitudes of the caregivers, the staffing patterns on the maternity unit, the policies and procedures followed by the caregivers, and the expectations of the professionals, as well as the expectations of the woman giving birth."[1]

In this chapter you will read about perspectives from clinicians who reveal how they view your pain during childbirth and how they will help you cope. You will read about:

- How caregivers are taught to respond to your labor pain.
- The birth plan and an evaluation of one hospital's birth plan log and its (not-so-surprising) results.
- How some caregivers feel distressed when women are in pain (even if the women themselves are managing just fine).
- The concern caregivers express for the laboring mom who arrives unprepared and frightened by her birth experience.
- Tips from your caregivers—for a joyful childbirth.

CHANGING ATTITUDES TOWARD YOUR PAIN

> **DID YOU KNOW?** *There is a commonly used expression among health care providers: "Pain is whatever the patient says it is." This axiom recognizes that pain is a subjective experience and that patients (not clinicians) should be regarded as the experts on their pain.*

In 2001, the national organization that gives accreditation to hospitals, known as the Joint Commission on Accreditation of Healthcare Organizations (JCAHO), called for the implementation of new standards for pain management nationwide. These standards are to be used for patients throughout the hospital who experience either acute (short-term), or chronic (long-term) pain.

This initiative has led to the promotion of a new approach to respond to the patient's experience of pain and an increased awareness that pain is often undertreated or ineffectively treated, at the expense of the patient's comfort.

DID YOU KNOW? *Studies that have evaluated how accurately caregivers assess their patients' pain levels have shown the caregivers' perceptions of pain were not consistent with the patients' own perceptions of pain. These studies have found that caregivers often* underestimate, *or* overestimate *pain levels and consistently do not provide adequate pain relief (analgesia).*[2]

We list a few of JCAHO's Standards Related to Pain Management for all patients in the hospital setting. These standards recognize that your caregivers should:

- Recognize the right of the patient to appropriate assessment and management of pain.
- Screen for the presence, and assess the nature and intensity of, pain in all patients.
- Determine and ensure staff competency in pain assessment and management.
- Establish policies and procedures that support the appropriate prescribing or ordering of pain medications.
- Educate patients and their families about the importance of effective pain management.[3]

IS YOUR CAREGIVER RATING YOUR PAIN LEVEL ACCURATELY?

To help ease your pain, your nurse or anesthesiologist must first understand how much pain you are experiencing. One simple strategy used throughout hospitals, and in labor and delivery units, is the use of a ten-point pain scale, with zero being "no pain" and ten being "the worst possible pain." You may be asked at various points throughout your labor, and throughout your recovery, "If you had to rate the pain you are feeling right now from one to ten, what number would you choose?" Your response helps your caregivers understand the intensity of the pain you are experiencing (if any) and allows you to decide together how to manage your comfort level.

Assessing your pain level and responding to meet your pain-management requests, however, is not always a straightforward process. Even with the use of pain-rating scales, there can sometimes be a disconnect between your pain level and your caregiver's perception of your pain level, which may result in your pain being underestimated. This disparity between how you experience pain and how your caregiver perceives your pain level can then lead to undertreatment of your pain. It is important that you communicate to your nurse, midwife, or anesthesiologist about how much pain or discomfort you are feeling, and ask for help in getting more comfortable.

On the other hand, some caregivers report that they may overestimate the laboring woman's need for pain relief when they see she is attempting to cope with her pain without the use of medications. This can lead to frustration on behalf of the laboring mom if she feels she is managing her pain adequately, but her caregivers, due to their own distress in dealing with a patient experiencing discomfort, respond by attempting to relieve her pain through the use of medications.

YOUR BIRTH PLAN—DOES ANYONE ACTUALLY READ IT?

A birth plan is simply a guideline you create to provide those who will be caring for you with an understanding of your preferences during your labor and birth experience. A birth plan typically addresses issues such as who you would like to have with you during labor and birth, what types of pain management and comfort measures you would prefer to try, and whether you would like to try to breast-feed right away after the birth of the baby.

Since your birth plan acts only as a guideline, you may change your mind at any time about preferences you have written in the plan. Any medically necessary action, of course, takes precedence over the preferences specified in the birth plan.

If you are interested in seeing examples of birth plans and learning more about how to create one for yourself, go to www.BirthPlan.com.

Depending on the circumstances and individuals involved, birth plans are sometimes welcomed as helpful tools used to better understand the wishes of the mother, and at other times they are dismissed as inflexible and entirely unrealistic. But take heart. Your birth plan does matter. In fact, the obstetric caregivers at Duke University Hospital in North Carolina saved two years' worth of women's birth plans and then studied them to identify what women want most during their birth experience. The trends revealed by the evaluation of the plans were then used by the hospital to consider implementation of changes designed to better meet the requests of their maternity patients.

DID YOU KNOW? *Out of a possible 150 requests made by moms-to-be, the top three requests to appear in the birth plans were:*

1. The ability to breast-feed immediately.
2. The availability of an epidural for pain relief during labor.
3. The participation of the father in the childbirth process (specific requests to cut the cord).[4]

We asked obstetric caregivers who are on the front lines at some of the busiest maternity units across the country to share their perspectives on the following issues concerning your labor pain:

- What is most important to *you* during childbirth.
- What it is like to work with women experiencing pain.

- Is there any "value" to your labor pain?
- What obstacles your caregivers deal with in the management of your labor pain.
- Whether pain relief (or pain) impacts your satisfaction with your birth experience.
- What makes for an "ideal" maternity patient and a "difficult" maternity patient?

Caregivers' Perspectives

Laura Goetzl, M.D. , an obstetrician and maternal-fetal medicine specialist at The Medical University of South Carolina, author of the book, *Conception and Pregnancy over 35*.

What Is Most Important to Women During Childbirth?

"I think women like to have a sense of control, even though this is hard to achieve, even for an obstetrician who is giving birth!"

What Is It Like Working with Women in Pain?

"The most important thing is to realize that women experience pain differently. Mostly, I try to keep lines of communication open so that I can understand how they perceive their pain and how they would like to treat it."

What Are Some Obstacles to the Management of Labor Pain?

"The thing that bothers me most is when we treat pain to make ourselves feel better. One classic example is giving women a medication called Phenergan with narcotics to make them more quiet, even though we know that it has little effect on pain. I also think that husbands deciding on pain relief for their wives is a problem."

Does Labor Pain Impact Women's Satisfaction with Their Childbirth Experience? Specifically, Does Less Pain Equal a More Satisfying Birth Experience?

"I don't think so. Women who have more pain can be just as satisfied. It all depends on their belief system."

Ananda Lowe, doula, Boston, Massachusetts, was the assistant director of the Association of Labor Assistants and Childbirth Educators (ALACE) for seven years

What are Some Obstacles to the Management of Labor Pain?

"Access to midwives and doulas is increasing, but many women still do not know that this option is available and that mothers report high satisfaction when they have a doula's support during childbirth. Lack of access and lack of public information is probably the largest obstacle."

Is There Value to Labor Pain?

"Yes, definitely. Labor pain gives important physiologic feedback to the mother about how to work with her own labor, to find the positions that will more quickly and comfortably facilitate giving birth to her baby."

Paula Schiavoni, R.N., a labor and delivery nurse at Crawford Long Hospital in Atlanta, Georgia

What Is Most Important to Women During Childbirth?

"A good outcome, a healthy baby. It is important to women to have their family around them. Each woman's desires are individual. Some women want no pain because they associate pain with disease or injury."

What Is It Like Working with Women in Pain?

"I don't mind it. If you educate the patient and help her understand the physiology of her pain, it helps to alleviate her anxiety. Then she can deal with and tolerate the pain. Nursing has a direct impact on the patient's perception of pain; you need to be constantly at her bedside during labor."

Describe the "Ideal" Maternity Patient

"Someone who is realistic in her expectations. A patient who can listen to what is going to be helpful for her to achieve a healthy outcome, who can understand what is happening to her body, is ideal."

Describe the "Difficult" Maternity Patient

"Women who are uneducated about what to expect during the childbirth process, and conversely, women who come in with a rigid birth plan and whose requests become unreasonable when a complication arises. Their refusal to allow for an IV or the use of other interventions can be frustrating when you feel they are putting themselves or their babies in an unsafe situation. There is nothing wrong with having a birth plan; I do love to work with women who are very educated about the birth process, have done their reading, and have a desire to treat childbirth as a normal, natural thing."

Barry J. Brock, M.D., an obstetrician, Beverly Hills, California

What Is Most Important to Women During Childbirth?

"First, women want to have a healthy labor experience. Second, they want to have a healthy, beautiful baby, and third, they want an enjoyable experience."

Is There Value to Labor Pain?

"Well, yes, it's a good clinical sign that they are about to have a baby! But, no, there is no advantage to experiencing severe pain."

Does Labor Pain Impact Women's Satisfaction with Their Childbirth Experience?

"Yes."

Specifically, Does Less Pain Equal a More Satisfying Birth?

"Yes. My patients can have an epidural anytime they want, even toward the end of labor. If they feel too numb to push, I taper off the medications, then when the baby begins to deliver, I have the epidural reactivated so they do not experience pain while pushing the baby out. This also provides an advantage to the mom if she needs to be sutured for a tear. In addition, it provides the benefit of good pain relief in the first few hours immediately after giving birth, which are often the most painful hours of recovery."

Ms. Theresa Lacey, R.N., a labor and delivery nurse for over twenty years at Duke University Medical Center, Durham, North Carolina

What Is Most Important to Women During Childbirth?

"I have never known a patient who was not afraid during her labor, even for repeat moms, sometimes especially for repeat moms, since they know what to expect. The nurse's physical presence is so important to help reduce their anxiety. Most patients want the simple things: listen to the radio, have her partner give her a back massage or be there to cut the umbilical cord. If you can accommodate women on a basic level, you can help put them at ease."

What Is It Like Working with Women in Pain?

"When I began over twenty-two years ago, there were very few epidurals given, so nurses and physicians had to develop other [nonmedical] techniques to help their patients. There is now a big generational shift, and nurses and physicians are no longer taught these techniques. It can be stressful to work with women in pain. Often clinicians become very anxious and want their patients to be medicated immediately due to their own anxiety. I understand how epidurals have become as popular as they have; they really do work and with not too much risk. But it is interesting to me that the younger nurses and doctors think it is miraculous when a woman actually gives birth without drugs!"

Is There Value to Labor Pain?

"There probably is value to labor pain, and there may be psychological benefits in the long run. That does not mean there is no value or benefit to being comfortable, if that is what you desire. You are no less of a woman or mother. I don't see the value in forcing a person to go through hours of excruciating pain. I wish that we were more balanced, though, that we could offer more options including the option of no medical pain relief."

Ingrid Carroll, R.N., a labor and delivery nurse manager in Atlanta, Georgia.

What Is Most Important to Women During Childbirth?

"Support and communication. Labor is such an unpredictable event that can change rapidly at any given time. I think women want to know that you are there for them, will listen to them, answer their questions, and guide them in the right direction. I think it is important for them to know that someone is watching over them."

Describe the "Ideal" Maternity Patient

"One who trusts health care professionals and keeps an open mind about her labor experience."

Describe the "Difficult" Maternity Patient

"Well, I hate to use the term *difficult* because a woman in pain is not herself. However, every so often you get that patient who distrusts the medical professionals, presumes all the nurses and doctors are only acting on their own agenda, and is determined that her labor is going to go a specific way."

Is There Value to Labor Pain?

"It serves a purpose; the body's functions that cause labor pain to occur are necessary to the process. But is there any value to women remaining in pain where there are safe options? That's a personal choice. Women choose whether to 'go natural' or opt for pain-relief measures."

Ho-Yu Pan, R.N., a labor and delivery nurse at Duke University Medical Center in Durham, North Carolina.

What Is Most Important to Women During Childbirth?

"Having their partner or support person with them throughout their labor process. They want no unnecessary separation from their baby. Women also want access to a full range of pain-management choices—in a timely fashion!"

What Is It Like Working with Women in Pain?

"It is very emotionally draining. A lot of work. It is not just about providing physical care; you are emotionally involved as well. But once you meet the patient's expectations, you feel the sunshine. It is important to honor your patients' pain and their expectation for pain management. If they say pain is ten out of ten on a rating scale, then that's what it is."

Describe the "Ideal" Maternity Patient

"The couple with an open mind who has a trusting relationship with their caregiver or provider is ideal. Women who try to labor with confidence. They may also experience fear, but confidence, too. They have some understanding of the labor process and realistic expectations. They are willing to try some nonpharmacological form of pain management to start with [such as breathing, relaxation, massage, aromatherapy] until they need medical pain management. I don't mind patients yelling or screaming. That does not make them 'difficult.'

"It is nice to work with a patient who knows her body and feels *she* has the power when she interacts with her caregiver. It is a great relationship when I am their support person and they are actively [not passively] interacting. Awesome!"

Describe the "Difficult" Maternity Patient

"One of two categories: First, the patient who does not trust her caregiver. I don't understand why they come to the hospital, when they have no trust whatsoever. Second, the couple who is hostile to current obstetric practices. Often they have the mind-set that the staff is going to control them, not allow freedom or the right to manage their own labor. It is difficult to deal with patients like that."

Is There Value to Labor Pain?

"Yes, I think so. The pain actually gives women a way to comfort themselves, by repositioning, taking a shower, asking for a massage, or other measures. By doing these things in response to her labor pain, she becomes more comfortable and will be able to get her baby in the optimal birth position."

Carolyn Ogren, R.N., and a certified doula, (DONA), in the Boston area

What Is Most Important to Women During Childbirth?
"Feeling cared for; feeling cared about and respected."

What Is It Like Working with Women in Pain?

"Initially it is frightening to work with women in pain, but with experience, it is rewarding since there are so many ways to help ease the physical and emotional pain, no matter what kind of labor and birth experience. The awe I feel as I witness the strength of each woman and the birth of a new family is still a special gift I receive, even after thirty-five years in the field."

Describe the "Ideal" Maternity Patient

"If 'ideal' means a patient I most enjoy working with, it would be someone who believes in herself and her ability to birth, and is amazed about the process and the experience; one who is open to support from others but, more important, listens to her body's wise messages. I also like to work with patients who have taken the responsibility and made the effort to become educated so that they make informed choices, whatever those choices may be."

Describe the "Difficult" Maternity Patient

"If difficult means evoking the most frustration in me, it would be someone who is not able to recognize that working together will make it better for her, someone with whom I cannot figure out how to connect on some personal level. A hostile patient is also hard to work with. I believe that this is usually because of immense fear, maybe due to lack of education about the process, lack of confidence in herself, or lack of trust in relationships."

Does Labor Pain Impact Women's Satisfaction with Their Childbirth Experience? Specifically, Does Less Pain Equal a More Satisfying Birth Experience?

"Yes, I do think that pain relief can impact a woman's experience, but I am not sure that it impacts her 'satisfaction,' if that means sense of accomplishment or being in control of her labor. No, I do not believe that less pain equals a more satisfying birth experience. I believe how her wishes are respected—

for example, receiving medication immediately when she requests it, or support when alternative methods are used, being
treated with dignity as an individual, and feeling cared about
(not being left alone, having a good, trusting relationship with
staff)—are all more important than the amount of pain she experiences."

Jill Noll, a certified nurse-midwife at Triangle Ob-Gyn in Cary, North Carolina

What Is Most Important to Women During Childbirth?
"The staff and the people who support the laboring woman
are most important. They help her make decisions that are right
for her. It is important for the support team to help women
with their wishes and not impose their own ideas on her."

Describe the "Ideal" Maternity Patient
"One who is open to all possibilities. Everyone's labor is different and there is no 'recipe' that is right for every woman."

Describe the "Difficult" Maternity Patient
"Someone who does not have trust in me or the establishment where they choose to deliver."

What Are Some Obstacles Concerning the Management of Labor Pain?
"I don't like the fact that the talk on the street is 'you have
to have an epidural . . . it's the only way to go . . . you're crazy
if you don't have an epidural.' I believe that every woman
should be able to have the birth that *she* wants, not the birth
that the doctor, nurse, nurse-midwife, husband, friend, book,
etc., thinks she should have."

Tips from Your Caregivers for a Childbirth with *Less Pain* and *More Joy*

The many perspectives and birth stories shared by caregivers of all disciplines boil down to a few commonsense observations regarding the topic of labor-pain relief. The simple suggestions or reminders they offer are based on years of experience in providing support to laboring women and can help you achieve the type of birth experience you desire, using the pain-management methods you prefer.

The Most Satisfied Mom on the Delivery Unit Is Prepared and Informed

Childbirth does not require an entrance exam, but a reasonable amount of preparation can go a long way toward helping you feel emotionally and physically comfortable throughout your labor and birth, especially given the often-unpredictable nature of childbirth. Caregivers agree that women who have an understanding of how their bodies work during childbirth, and have basic information about their birth environment and their pain-management options, are more likely to have a satisfying birth experience, even if it turns out to be entirely unlike what they had anticipated.

Trust Your Caregivers and Let Them Give You Care

You should be able to trust that your caregiver is in sync with your birth preferences and will provide you with good support throughout your labor and birth. In the heat of labor, this may require a leap of faith, but if you are both "on the same page" regarding your pain-management choices, you may need to let your caregiver take the lead. That said . . .

Trust Yourself

Caregivers have repeatedly observed that women who have confidence in their own ability to give birth—regardless of the method of pain management they choose—women who can clearly request (not demand) their preferences in the labor and delivery unit—and see their births as something they are doing, not something the staff is doing for them, consistently have a more satisfying birth experience.

Be Flexible

Caregivers throughout these chapters have stated, in one way or another, the importance of being flexible in your birth plan, as your labor progresses. This does not imply that you should necessarily depart from your original plan. But, it does suggest that in the face of an unplanned event (for example, a labor that moves more quickly than you had anticipated), remaining flexible with your pain-management plans—regardless of the type of plan—will help you deal with whatever comes your way during labor and delivery, and help you achieve a positive birth experience. Remaining flexible also allows you to feel fine *after* you give birth, rather than regretful for not experiencing the exact childbirth scenario you had planned on.

We Have a Shared Goal: A Positive Birth Experience and a Healthy Baby

You may have noticed, whether the caregiver is an anesthesiologist providing medical pain relief all day long, or a doula who specializes in waterbirth—regardless of birth philosophy or pain-management techniques used by labor professionals—the goal is always the same: to ensure the safe birth of a healthy baby and to provide you with a comfortable birth experience filled with *less pain* and *more joy*.

Notes

CHAPTER ONE

1. World Health Organization (1997). *Care in Normal Birth: A Practical Guide,* p. 16. (Geneva: World Health Organization).

2. BA Bucklin, M.D., JL Hawkins, M.D., JR Anderson, Ph.D., FA Ullrich, B.A., Obstetric Anesthesia Workforce Survey, Twenty-Year Update, *Anesthesiology,* v 103, No 3, Sept 2005;: 645–53.

3. Maternity Center Association (October 2002). Listening to Mothers: Report of the First National U.S. Survey of Women's Childbearing Experiences. Executive Summary and Recommendations Issued by the Maternity Center Association (New York: Maternity Center Association).

4. National Association of Childbearing Centers; www.birthcenters.org.

5. JP Rooks, NL Weatherby, EK Ernst, S Stapleton, D Rosen, and A Rosenfield (December 1989). Outcomes of care in birth centers: The National Birth

Center Study. *The New England Journal of Medicine* 321(26):1804–11.

6. Ibid.

7. Maternity Center Association (October 2002).

8. Family Centered Maternity and Newborn Care: National Guideline (2005). Reproduced with the permission of the Minister of Public Works and Government Services Canada. (Ottawa, Health Canada, 2002).

9. Ed Hodnett (May 2002). Pain and women's satisfaction with the experience of childbirth: a systematic review. *American Journal of Obstetrics and Gynecology,* 186 (5) (Suppl)): S160–72.

CHAPTER TWO

1. American College of Obstetricians and Gynecologists (July 2004). Pain relief during labor. *Obstetrics and Gynecology* 104:213.

2. *American Baby* magazine; www.americanbaby.com.

3. P Simkin (June 1992). Just another day in a woman's life? Part II: Nature and consistency of women's long-term memories of their first birth experiences. *Birth* 19(2):64–81.

4. E Norwitz, JNA Robinson, and JRG Challis (August 1999). The control of labor. *The New England Journal of Medicine* 341(9):660–66.

5. Ibid.

6. CL Pasero and R Britt (August 1998). Managing pain during labor. *American Journal of Nursing* 98:10–11.

7. R Melzack, P Taenzer, P Feldman, and RA Kinch (1981). Labour is still painful after prepared childbirth training. *Canadian Medical Association Journal* 125:357–63.

8. Maternity Center Association (October 2002). Listening to Mothers: Report of the First National U.S. Survey of Women's Childbearing Experiences. Executive Summary and Recommendations Issued by the Maternity Center Association (New York: Maternity Center Association); www.maternitywise.org.

9. N Lowe (May 2002). The nature of labor pain. *American Journal of Obstetrics and Gynecology* 186(5)(Suppl):S16–S24.

10. M Wuitchik, K Hesson, and D Bakal (December 1990). Perinatal predictors of pain and distress during labor. *Birth* 17(4):186–91.

11. F Gerd and F Gaston-Johansson (1990). Do primiparas and multiparas have realistic expectations of labor? *Obstetricia et Gynecologica Scandinavica* 69:103–09.

12. J Alexander, S Sharma, D McIntire, J Wiley, and K Leveno (2001). Intensity of labor pain and cesarean delivery. *Anesthesia Analgesia* 92:1524–28.

13. R Melzack and E Belanger (1989). Labour pain: Correlations with menstrual pain and acute low-back pain before and during pregnancy. *Pain* 36:225–29.

14. PE Hess, TP Luca, SD Pratt, AK Soni, T Corbett, CG Miller, MC Sarna, and NE Oriol (April 1999). Oxytocin produces more painful labor. *Anesthesiology* 90(4AS)(Suppl):64A.

15. R Melzack, E Belanger, and R Lacroix (November 1991). Labor pain: Effect of maternal position on front and back pain. *Journal of Pain and Symptom Management* 6(8):476–80.

16. NK Lowe (May 2002).

17. Ibid.

18. R Melzack, P Taenzer, P Feldman, and RA Kinch (August 1981).

CHAPTER THREE

1. S Bewley and J Cockburn (June 2002). Responding to fear of childbirth. *The Lancet* 359:2128–29.

2. S Alehagen, K Wijma, and B Wijma (April 2001). Fear during labor. *Acta Obstetricia et Gynecologica Scandinavica* 80(4):315.

3. H-L Melender (June 2002). Experiences of fears associated with pregnancy and childbirth: A study of 329 pregnant women. *Birth* 29(2):101.

4. National Center for Health Statistics (January 2002). Explaining the 2001–2002 Infant Mortality Increase: Data From the Linked Birth/Infant Death Data Set, *National Vital Statistics Reports,* Vol. 53, No. 12.

5. J Chang, LD Elam-Evans, CJ Berg, J Herndon, L Flowers, KA Seed, and CJ Syverson. Division of Reproductive Health, National Center for Chronic Disease Prevention and Health Promotion (February 2003). Pregnancy related mortality surveillance. *Morbidity and Mortality Weekly Report,* US 1991–1999. 52(2):1–8.

6. World Health Organization (2004). Maternal Mortality in 2000. Estimates developed by WHO, UNICEF, and UNFPA. Department of Reproductive Health and Research (Geneva: World Health Organization).

7. K Hofberg and I Brockington (2000). Tokophobia: An unreasoning dread of childbirth. *British Journal of Psychiatry* 176:83–85.

8. T Saisto and E Halmesmaki (March 2003). Fear of childbirth: A neglected dilemma. *Acta Obstetricia et Gynecologica Scandinavica* 82(3):201–08.

9. T Saisto, O Yiikorkala, and E Halmesmaki (November 1999). Factors associated with fear of delivery in second pregnancies. *Obstetrics and Gynecology* 94(5):679–82.

10. Ibid.

11. Ibid.

12. S Bewley and J Cockburn (June 2002). Responding to the fear of childbirth. *The Lancet* 359(9324):2128–29.

13. M Lobel (2004) Pregnancy. In AJ Christensen, R Martin & JM Smyth (eds.). *Encyclopedia of Health Psychology* (New York: Kluwer Academic/Plenum).

14. Y Rofe, M Blittner, and I Lewin (January 1993). Emotional experiences during three trimesters of pregnancy. *Journal of Clinical Psychology* (1):3–12.

15. IS Federenko and PD Wadhwa (March 2004). Women's mental health during pregnancy influences fetal and

infant development and health outcomes. *CNS Spectrums* 9(3):198–206.

16. D Armstrong and M Hutti (March–April 1998). Pregnancy after perinatal loss: The relationship between anxiety and prenatal attachment. *Journal of Obstetric, Gynecologic and Neonatal Nursing* 27(2):183–89.

17. A Gupton, M Heaman, and T Ashcroft (July–August 1997). Bed rest from the perspective of the high-risk pregnant woman. *Journal of Obstetric, Gynecologic and Neonatal Nursing* 26(4):423–30.

18. JC Campbell (May 2001). Abuse during pregnancy: A quintessential threat to maternal and child health—So when do we start to act? *Canadian Medical Association Journal* 164(11):1578–79.

19. P Simkin (1992). Overcoming the legacy of childhood sexual abuse: The role of caregivers and childbirth educators. *Birth* 19:224–25.

20. T Hampton (September 2004). Fetal environment may have profound long-term consequences for health. *Journal of the American Medical Association* 292(11):1285–86.

21. J McCubbin, E Lawson, S Cox, J Sherman, J Norton, and J Read (September 1996). Prenatal maternal blood pressure response to stress predicts birthweight and gestational age: A pregnancy study. *American Journal of Obstetrics and Gynecology* 175(3):706–12.

CHAPTER FOUR

1. C Wong, B Scavone, A Peaceman, R McCarthy, J Sullivan, N Diaz, E Yaghmour, R-J Marcus, Sherwani, M Sproviero, M Yilmaz, R Patel, C Robles, and S Grouper (February 2005). The risk of cesarean delivery with neuraxial analgesia given early versus late in labor. *The New England Journal of Medicine* 352(7):655–65. See also A Vahratian, J Zhang, J Hasling, et al. (2004). The effect of early epidural versus early intravenous analgesia use on labor

progression: A natural experiment. *American Journal of Obstetrics and Gynecology* 191:259–65.

2. S Torvaldsen, C Roberts, J Bell, and C Raynes-Greenow (October 18, 2004). Discontinuation of epidural analgesia late in labour for reducing the adverse delivery outcomes associated with epidural analgesia. *The Cochrane Database of Systematic Reviews* 4:CD004457.

3. BL Leighton and SH Halpern (May 2002). The effects of epidural analgesia on labor, maternal and neonatal outcomes: A systematic review. *American Journal of Obstetrics and Gynecology* 186(5):S69–S77.

4. Y Beilin, J Zahn, HH Bernstein, B Zucker-Pinchoff, WJ Zenzen, and LA Andres (June 1998).Treatment of incomplete analgesia after placement of an epidural catheter and administration of local anesthetic for women in labor. *Anesthesiology* 88(6):1502–6.

5. Leighton and Halpern (May 2002).

6. JL Hawkins, LM Koonin, SK Palmer, and CP Gibbs (February 1997). Anesthesia-related deaths during obstetric delivery in the United States, 1979–1990. *Anesthesiology* 86(2):277–84.

7. Leighton and Halpern (May 2002).

8. S Sharma, D McIntire, J Wiley, and K Leveno (2004). Labor analgesia and cesarean delivery: An individual patient meta-analysis of nulliparous women. *Anesthesiology* 100:142–48.

9. M Wuitchik, D Bakal, and J Lipshitz (1989). The clinical significance of pain and cognitive activity in latent labor. *Obstetrics and Gynecology* 73:35–42.

10. PE Hess, SD Pratt, AK Soni, MC Sarna, and NE Oriol (2002). An association between severe labor pain and cesarean delivery. *Anesthesia Analgesia* 90:881–86.

11. S Segal, M Su, and P Gilbert (October 2000). The effect of rapid change in availability of epidural analgesia on the cesarean delivery rate: A meta-analysis.

American Journal of Obstetrics and Gynecology 183(4): 974–78.

12. S Segal, R Blatman, M Doble, and S Datta (July 1999). The influence of the obstetrician in the relationship between epidural analgesia and cesarean section for dystocia. *Anesthesiology* 91(1):90–96.

13. W Howell (1999). Epidural versus non-epidural analgesia for pain relief in labour (2003). *The Cochrane Database of Systematic Reviews* 3:CD000331.

14. HK Eltzschig, ES Lieberman, and WR Camann (January 23, 2003). Regional anesthesia and analgesia for labor and delivery. *The New England Journal of Medicine* 348(4):319–32. See also PJ Alexander, SK Sharma, KJ Leveno, DD McIntire, and J Wiley (May 1999). Epidural analgesia during labor and maternal fever. *Anesthesiology* 90(5):1271–75.

15. L Goetzl, A Cohen, F Frigoletto Jr, SA Ringer, JM Lang, and E Lieberman (November 2001). Maternal epidural use and neonatal sepsis evaluation in afebrile mothers. *Pediatrics* 108(5):1099–1102.

16. JH Charlotte, T Dean, L Lucking, K Dziedzic, PW Jones, and RB Johanson (August 17, 2002). Randomised study of long-term outcome after epidural versus non-epidural analgesia during labour. *British Medical Journal* 325(7360):357.

17. Sharma et al. (January 2004).

18. S Segal et al. (July 1999).

19. AH Shennan and Comparative Obstetric Mobile Epidural Trial (COMET) Study Group UK (July 2002). Effect of low-dose mobile versus traditional epidural techniques on mode of delivery: A randomised controlled trial. *The Lancet* 358(9275):19–23.

20. Sharma et al. (January 2004).

21. J Zhang, MK Yancy, MA Klebanoff, J Schwarz, and D Schwitzer (July 2001). Does epidural analgesia prolong labor and increase risk of cesarean delivery? A

natural experiment. *American Journal of Obstetrics and Gynecology* 185(1):128–34.

22. M Kubli, MJ Scrutton, PT Seed, and G O'Sullivan (February 2002). An evaluation of isotonic "sport drinks" during labor. *Anesthesia Analgesia* 94(2):404–08.

23. SH Halpern, T Levine, WB Wilson, J MacDonell, SE Katsiris, and BL Leighton (December 1999). Effect of labor analgesia on breastfeeding success. *Birth* 26(4):275–76.

24. A Albani, P Addamo, A Renghi, G Voltolin, L Peano, and G Ivani (1999). The effect on breastfeeding rate of regional anesthesia technique for cesarean and vaginal childbirth. *Minerva Anesthesiology* 6:25–30.

25. AD Sia, WR Camann, CE Ocampo, RW Goy, HM Tan, and S Rajammal (2003). Neuraxial block for labour analgesia: Is the combined spinal epidural (CSE) modality a good alternative to conventional analgesia? *Singapore Medical Journal* 44(9):464–70. See also Eltzschig, Lieberman, and Camann (January 23, 2003).

26. Sia et al. (2003).

27. D Hughes, SW Simmons, J Brown, and AM Cyna (2003). Combined spinal-epidural versus epidural analgesia in labour. *The Cochrane Database of Systematic Reviews* 4:CD003401.

28. ES Ledin, C Gentele, and CH Olofsson (October 2003). PCEA compared to continuous epidural infusion in an ultra-low-dose regimen for labor-pain relief: A randomized study. *Acta Anaesthesiologica Scandinavica* 47(9):1085–90.

29. M van der Vyver, S Halpern, and G Joseph (2002). Patient-controlled epidural analgesia versus continuous infusion for labour analgesia: A meta-analysis. *British Journal of Anaesthesia* 89:459–65.

CHAPTER FIVE

1. JL Hawkins, BR Beaty, and CP Gibbs (1999). Update on obstetric anesthesia practices in the U.S. *Anesthesiology* 91:1060.

2. BL Leighton and S Halpern (2002). The effects of epidural analgesia on labor, maternal, neonatal outcomes: A systematic review. *American Journal of Obstetrics and Gynecology* 186:S69–S77.

3. DH Chestnut (2004). Parenteral and inhalational agents. In DH Chestnut (ed.), *Obstetric Anesthesia Principles and Practice,* 3rd ed., pp. 311–23 (Philadelphia: Elsevier Mosby).

4. Ibid.

5. Ibid.

6. Ibid.

7. WE Rayburn, CV Smith, JD Parriott, and RE Woods (October 1989). Randomized comparison of meperidine and fentanyl during labor. *Obstetrics and Gynecology* 74(4):604–06.

8. C Wilson, E McClean, J Moore, and JW Dundee (December 1986). A double-blind comparison of intramuscular pethidine and nalbuphine in labour. *Anaesthesia* 41(12):1207–13.

9. E Nissen, AM Widstrom, G Lilja, AS Matthiesen, K Uvnal-Moberk, G Jacobsson, and LO Boreus (February 1997). Effects of routinely given pethidine during labour on infants' developing breast-feeding behaviour: Effects of dose-delivery time interval and various concentrations of pethidine/norpethidine in cord plasma. *Acta Paediatrica* 86(2): 201–28.

CHAPTER SIX

1. Lamaze International; www.lamaze-childbirth.com.

2. Ibid.

3. Ibid.

4. Ibid.

5. Ibid.

6. Ibid.

7. American Academy of Husband-Coached Childbirth; www.bradleybirth.com.

8. Global Maternal Child Health Association; www.waterbirth.org.

9. ER Cluett, VC Nikodem, RE McCandlish, and EE Burns (2004). Immersion in water in pregnancy, labour and birth. *The Cochrane Database of Systematic Reviews* 2:CD000111.

10. H Richmond (March 2003). Women's experience of waterbirth. *The Practicing Midwife* 6(3):26–31.

11. RE Gilbert and PA Tookey (August 1999). Perinatal mortality and morbidity among babies delivered in water: Surveillance study and postal survey. *British Medical Journal* 21(319):483–87.

12. CM Otigbah, MK Ohanjal, G Harmsworth, and T Chard (July 2002). A retrospective comparison of waterbirths and conventional vaginal deliveries. *European Journal of Obstetric and Gynecological Reproduction Biology* 91(1):15–20.

13. S Pellantova, Z Vebera, and P Pucek (January 2003). Water delivery: A five-year retrospective study. *Ceskoslovenska Gynekologie* 68(3):175–79.

14. V Geissbuhler and J Eberhard (September–October 2000). Waterbirths: A comparative study. A prospective study on more than 2,000 waterbirths. *Fetal Diagnosis and Therapy* 15(5):291–300.

15. E Cluett, R Pickering, K Getliffe, and NJ St George Saunders (February 7, 2004). Randomised controlled trial of labouring in water compared with standard of augmentation for management of dystocia in first stage of labour. *British Medical Journal* 328(7435):314.

16. VC Nicodem (2000). Immersion in water in pregnancy, labour and birth. *The Cochrane Database of Systematic Reviews* 2:CD000111.

17. A Cyna, G McAuliffe, and M Andrew (2004). Hypnosis for pain relief in labour and childbirth: A systematic review. *British Journal of Anaesthesia* 93(4):505–11.

18. A Ewies and K Olah (March 2002). Moxibustion in

breech version: A descriptive review. *Acupuncture Medicine* 20(1):26–29. See also I Neri, G Airola, G Contu, G Allais, F Facchinetti, and C Benedetto (April 2004). Acupuncture plus moxibustion to resolve breech presentation: A randomized controlled study. *Journal of Maternal and Fetal Neonatal Medicine* 15(4):247–52.

19. CA Smith, CT Collins, AM Cyna, and CA Crowther (2003). Complementary and alternative therapies for pain management in labour. *The Cochrane Database of Systematic Reviews 2:* CD003521.

20. ED Hodnett, S Gates, GJ Hofmeyr, and C Sakala (2004). Continuous support for women during childbirth. *The Cochrane Database of Systematic Reviews 2:* CD003766.

21. ED Hodnett, NK Lowe, ME Hannah, AR Willan, B Stevens, JA Weston, A Ohlsson, A Gafni, H Muir, TL Myhr, and R Stremler (September 18, 2002). Effectiveness of nurses as providers of birth labor support in North American hospitals. *The Journal of the American Medical Association* 288(11):1373–81.

22. EE Burns, C Blamey, SJ Ersser, et al. (2000). An investigation into the use of aromatherapy in intrapartum midwifery practice. *Journal of Alternative and Complementary Medicine* 6:141–47.

23. L Martensson, K Nyberg, G Wallin (2002). Subcutaneous versus intracutaneous injections of sterile water for labour analgesia: a comparison of perceived pain during administration. *British Journal of Obstetrics and Gynaecology* 107 (10): 1248–1251.

24. JL Reynolds (March 2000). In the literature: Sterile water injections relieve back pain of labor. *Birth* 27(1):58.

25. T Lytzen, L Cederberg, and J Moller-Nielsen (1989). Relief of low back pain in labor by using intracutaneous nerve stimulation (INS) with sterile

water papules. *Acta Obstetricia et Gynecologica Scandinavica* 68(4):341–43.

26. B Kaplan, D Rabinerson, S Lurie, J Bar, UR Krieser, and A Neri (March 1988). Transcutaneous electrical nerve stimulation TENS for adjuvant relief during labour and delivery. *International Journal of Gynaecology and Obstetrics* 60(3):251–55.

27. D Carroll, RA Moore, MR Tramer, and HJ McQuay (February 1997). Transcutaneous electrical nerve stimulation does not relieve labour pain: Updated systematic review. *British Journal of Obstetrics and Gynaecology* 104(2):169–75.

CHAPTER SEVEN

1. National Center for Health Statistics September 2005. Births—Method of Delivery (Data for United States in 2003), U.S. Department of Health and Human Service Centers for Disease Control and Prevention; www.cdc.gov.

2. P Choi, S Galinski, L Takeuchi, S Lucas, C Tamayo, and A Jadad (2003). PDPH is a common complication of neuraxial blockade in parturients: A meta-analysis of obstetrical studies. *Canadian Journal of Anesthesia* 50:460–69.

3. U Aromaa, M Lahdensuu, and DA Cozanitis (April 1997). Severe complications associated with epidural and spinal anaesthesias in Finland 1987–1993: A study based on patient insurance claims. *Acta Anaesthesiologica Scandinavica* 41(4):445–52.

4. JL Hawkins, LM Koonin, SK Palmer, and CP Gibbs (1997). Anesthesia-related deaths during obstetric delivery in the United States, 1979–1990. *Anesthesiology* 86:277.

5. G Briggs, RK Freeman, and SJ Yaffe (1994). *Drugs in Pregnancy and Lactation,* 4th ed., p. 651 (Baltimore: Williams & Wilkins).

6. American Academy of Pediatrics (September 2001).

The transfer of drugs and other chemicals into human milk. Policy statement. *Pediatrics* 108(3)776–89.

CHAPTER EIGHT

1. HM Schaer (1980). History of pain relief in obstetrics. In GF Marx and GM Bassell (eds.). *Obstetric Analgesia and Anesthesia*, pp. 1–19 (Amsterdam: Elsevier/North Holland, Biomedical Press).

2. V French (1986). Midwives and maternity care in the Roman world. *Helios, New Series* 13(2):69–84.

3. PP Sim (September 1997). "To give birth without pain!": The first cases of mesmeric pain relief for obstetrics. *American Society of Anesthesiologists* 61(9):14–16.

4. LS Euphenia Maclean (2004). Agnes Sampson, and pain relief in 16th-century Edinburgh. *Anaesthesia* 59:834–5.

5. D Caton (1999). *What a Blessing She Had Chloroform: The Medical and Social Response to the Pain of Childbirth from 1800 to the Present*, pp. 104–07 (New Haven, CT: Yale University Press).

6. R Clark, F Longfellow, and N Keep (September 1997). *American Society of Anesthesiologists Newsletter* 16(9).

7. AS Williams (1997). *Women and Childbirth in the Twentieth Century: A History of the National Birthday Trust Fund 1928–93,* p. 143 (Stroud, England: Sutton Publishing).

8. Caton (1999), p. 139.

9. Ibid., pp. 162–71.

10. Ibid., p. 160.

11. AS Williams (1997). *Women and Childbirth in the Twentieth Century: A History of the National Birthday Trust Fund 1928–93,* p. 1 (Stroud, England: Sutton Publishing).

12. JL Hawkins, BR Beaty, and C Gibbs (1999). Update on obstetric anesthesia practices in the U.S. *Anesthesiology* 91: A1060.

CHAPTER ELEVEN

1. Family Centered Maternity and Newborn Care: National Guidelines (2005). Reproduced with the permission of the Minister of Public Works and Government Services Canada (Ottawa: Health Canada, 2000).

2. E Sheiner, R Hershkovits, M Mazor, M Katz, and I Shoham-Vardi (2000). Overestimation and underestimation of labor pain. *European Journal of Obstetrics and Gynecology and Reproductive Biology* 91:37–40.

3. 2000–2001 Joint Commission on Accreditation of Healthcare Organizations. PAIN: Current understanding of assessment management and treatments. Strategies to improve pain management. *Standards Manual,* pp. 77–78.

4. A Olufolabi and H Pan (2004). Birth plans: What is important to the laboring parturient? *Anesthesiology* 100(Supp 1):48.

Further Acknowledgments

We would like to thank the many professionals who provided valuable contributions to this book, through interviews, direct quotes, birth-case scenarios, and their own personal birth stories.

Thank you to the following individuals for providing interesting case scenarios and advice to our readers on how to ensure their pain management plans do not go awry: Mark Zakowski, M.D., chief of obstetric anesthesia, Cedars–Sinai Hospital, Los Angeles, California; Ann Rehm, M.D., obstetrician and gynecologist, William Beaumont Hospital, Royal Oak, Michigan; Gerry Bassell, M.D., obstetric anesthesiologist, Wesley Medical Center, Wichita, Kansas; Gayle Riedmann, certified nurse-midwife, Oak Park, Illinois; Robyn Faye, M.D., obstetrician, Mercy Suburban Hospital, Norristown, Pennsylvania.

We especially appreciate the contributions from the obstetric professionals who allowed us to share their personal birth stories with our readers: Kathryn Zuspan, M.D., obstetric anesthesiologist, Lakeview Hospital, Stillwater, Minnesota; Rachel Dolan Wickersham, certified doula, Chicago, Illinois;

Suzan Ulrich, certified nurse-midwife, chair of midwifery and women's health, Frontier School of Midwifery and Family Nursing; Cynthia Wong, M.D., director of obstetric anesthesiology, Northwestern University Feinberg School of Medicine, Chicago, Illinois; Lauren Streicher, M.D., obstetrician/gynecologist and journalist, Chicago, Illinois; Medge Owen, M.D., anesthesiologist, associate professor of obstetric anesthesiology, Wake Forest University, Winston-Salem, North Carolina.

Our thanks to the following people, who provided us with their point of view about how women deal with their labor pain, and shared their candid comments about the emotional aspects of labor pain and labor-pain relief: Laura Goetzl, M.D., obstetrician and maternal-fetal medicine specialist, The Medical University of South Carolina, South Carolina; Ananda Lowe, doula, Boston, Massachusetts; Paula Schiavoni, R.N., Crawford Long Hospital, Atlanta, Georgia; Barry J. Brock, M.D., obstetrician, Beverly Hills, California; Theresa Lacey, R.N., Duke University Medical Center, North Carolina; Ingrid Carroll, R.N., Atlanta, Georgia; Ho-Yu Pan, R.N., Duke University Medical Center, North Carolina; Carolyn Ogren, R.N., certified doula, Boston, Massachusetts; Jill Knoll, certified nurse-midwife, Triangle Ob-Gyn, Cary, North Carolina.

Our gratitude to the following professionals, who shared their wisdom on the topic of labor pain and provided advice to readers on how they can and should prepare themselves for a positive birth experience: Debbie Pickens, R.N., Parkland Memorial Hospital, Dallas, Texas; Lisa Walsh, certified nurse-midwife, Women's Health Care, Anna Jaques Hospital, Newburyport, Massachusetts; Marcia Patterson, R.N., Rush Presbyterian St. Luke's Medical Center, Chicago, Illinois; Diedre A. Dibal, certified nurse-midwife, Bethany Women's Care, Kansas City, Kansas; Julia Lange Kessler, certified midwife, HVO Midwives, Nyack Hospital, New York; Tracey Hartley, certified doula, B★E★S★T Doula Service, Los Angeles, California; Ronald Ramus, M.D., obstetrician, Parkland Memorial Hospital, Dallas, Texas; T. Bogard, M.D., obstetric anesthesiologist, Wake

Forest University School of Medicine and Forsyth Medical Center, Winston-Salem, North Carolina.

Thank you to the experts who provided our readers with insight into the psychological aspects of pregnancy and childbirth, Diana Dell, M.D., obstetrician and psychiatrist, Duke University, North Carolina; James McCubbin, Ph.D., professor and chair of psychology, Clemson University, South Carolina; Marci Lobel, Ph.D., associate professor and director of Stony Brook Pregnancy Project, at Stony Brook University, New York.

Thank you also to all of the childbirth experts who reviewed our work for accuracy, or provided us with their expertise (and were generous with their time) by phone and e-mail: Errol Norwitz, M.D., Ph.D., director of perinatal research and associate director, Division of Maternal-Fetal Medicine, Yale University School of Medicine; Donald Caton, M.D., professor emeritus Departments of Anesthesiology and Obstetrics and Gynecology, University of Florida College of Medicine, Gainesville, Florida; Joy Hawkins, M.D., obstetric anesthesiologist, University of Colorado; Penny Simkin, P.T., certified doula, co-founder of DONA International, Valerie Arkoosh, M.D., obstetric anesthesiologist, David Birnbach, M.D., chief of women's anesthesia, University of Miami; James Eisenach, professor of anesthesiology, Wake Forest University Baptist Medical Center; Maureen Connolly and Dana Sullivan, authors of *The Essential C-Section Guide;* Robbie-Davis Floyd, Ph.D., Senior Research Fellow, Department of Anthropology, University of Texas, Austin; Barbara Harper, R.N., founder of Waterbirth International; Nancy Lowe, Ph.D., CNM, Oregon Health and Science University; Nancy Wainer Cohen, CPM, CCE; Kerry Tuschhoff, HCHI, CHt, founder of Hypnobabies, and many others in the field, thank you.

Our gratitude to all of the professionals from each of the different birth approaches, who allowed us to hear your point of view and provided our readers with expertise directly from the source: Holly Muir, M.D., chief of women's anesthesiology, Duke University Health System, North Carolina; Mark Rosen, M.D., anesthesiologist, University of California, San Francisco, California; Felicity Plaat, M.D., anesthesiologist, Queen Charlotte's Hospital, London; Biddy Fein, certified nurse-midwife, Brigham and Women's Hospital, Boston, Massachusetts; Linda Harmon, executive director, Lamaze International; Laura Conrad, certified Bradley instructor, North Carolina; Brooke Arnold, Doula and CPM; Bebe Amour, Inc., Dallas, Texas; Valerie Hobbs, associate professsor, South West Acupuncture College, Boulder, Colorado; Marsha Connor, R.N., OMD, Los Angeles, California; Jane Look, certified doula, Boston, Massachusetts; Nancy Wiand, R.N., Robinson Memorial Hospital, Ravenna, Ohio; Jude Stensland, nurse-midwife, Margie Bissinger, physical therapist, New Jersey; Polly Perez, R.N., doula, Johnson, Vermont.

And, finally, we are indebted to all of the women whom we interviewed over the last two years, who freely shared with us one of the most intimate and powerful moments of their lives, often providing extreme detail on the emotional and physical aspects of their labor and birth experiences. Your birth stories, whether beautiful or harrowing, helped guide the direction of this book, and provided our readers with an honest point of view from the other experts—the moms. To all of the moms who are quoted in this book, and the many others who shared their birth stories with us, thank you.

William Camann and Kathryn J. Alexander

Index

abuse
  domestic or emotional as stress
    factor, 67
acetaminophen
  pain relief and breast-feeding after
    cesarean delivery, 212
acupuncture, 140, 175–80
  caregiver's perspective, 179
  conditions or situations that would
    prevent use, 178
  how it is done and feels, 176
  moxibustion, 177
  partner's role, 177
  potential benefits, 178
  potential limitations, 178
  potential side effects, 178
  reasons for choosing, 176
  resources, 179–80
  what it is and does, 175–76
  when to use, 177
alternative approaches. *See*
    complementary and alternative
    approaches
American Academy of Family
    Physicians, 20

American Academy of Husband-
    Coached Childbirth, 153–54
American Academy of Pediatrics,
    212
American Association of Nurse
    Anesthetists, 17
American Association of Oriental
    Medicine, 179
American Baby magazine, 26
American College of Nurse-
    Midwives, 19, 181
American College of Obstetricians
    and Gynecologists (ACOG), 13,
    25
American Society of
    Anesthesiologists, 17
analgesics, 124–27
  Demerol (Meperidine), 125
  Fentanyl, 126
  Morphine, 125–26
  Nubain (Nalbuhine), 126
  potential benefits, 124
  potential side effects, 126–27
  potential side effects on baby, 127
  Stadol (Butorphanol), 126

analgesics (*cont.*)
  what you may feel, 122
  when to use, 124
anesthesia (timeline), 219–28
  1800s (James Young Simpson), 219
  1853 (Queen Victoria inhales
    chloroform gas), 221–22
  1847 (first American to use), 220
  early 1900s (women's political
    struggle), 220–22
  1914 (National Twilight Sleep
    Association), 222–24
  1940s–1970s (natural child-birth),
    225–27
  1980s–1990s (epidural becomes
    popular), 227
  2000s (blending of both sides),
    227–28
anesthesiologist, 1517
anesthetic. *See* local anesthetic agents
Apgar, Virginia, 90
Arnold, Brooke, 162
aromatherapy, 140, 185–91
  caregiver's perspective, 190
  essential oils used, 186–87
  how it is done and feels, 186–87
  partner's role, 188
  potential benefits, 188–89
  potential limitations, 189
  research says, 189
  resources, 191
  when to use, 187–88
aspirin
  pain relief and breast-feeding after
    cesarean delivery, 212
assisted delivery. *See* instrumental
    delivery
Association of Labor Assistants and
    Childbirth Educators (ALACE),
    23, 185
Association of Women's Health
    Obstetric and Neonatal Nurses
    (AWHONN), 15

back labor, 31
Bassell, Dr. Gerry, 235

bed rest
  high-risk pregnancy and 66–67
Bell, Kimberly G., 151–52
bergamot, 187
birth ball, 141, 197–99
  caregiver's perspective, 199
  how it is done and feels, 197
  partner's role, 198
  potential benefits, 198
  potential limitations, 198
  resources, 199
  what it is and does, 197
  when to use, 198
*Birth Ball: The Physical Therapy Balls
    in Maternity Care* (Perez), 199
birth center, 7–12
  hospital, transfer to, 9
  pro and cons, 10–12
  reasons to choose, 8–9
  satisfaction rate, 9
*Birth Partner: Everything You Need to
    Know to Help a Woman Through
    Childbirth, The* (Simkin), 185
birth plan, 272–74
  subject to change, 233–35
birth stories (from medical
    practitioners), 229–45
  birth plan, subject to change,
    233–35
  education as key, 243–45
  realistic expectations, flexible
    plans, 235–39
  same goal in mind, 230–32
  "what-ifs," preparing for,
    239–42
birth stories (from medical
    practitioners as patients),
    246–68
  from general anesthesia to epidural
    at home, 250–55
  an introduction, an epidural, a
    baby, 255–58
  Hollywood delivery, 247–50
  not afraid just curious, 264–68
  wait and see, 258–61
  when plans go wrong, 261–64
birthing stool, 217

bloodletting (leeches)
  as pain relief, 217
Bogard, Dr. T., 50
Bradley Method, 140, 147–54
  caregiver's perspective, 149–50
  potential benefits, 149
  potential limitations, 149
  reasons for choosing, 148
  resources, 153–54
  what it is and does, 147–48
  what women say, 149–54
Bradley, Dr. Robert A., 147, 226–27
breast-feeding
  pain relief after cesarean delivery,
    212
Brock, Dr. Barry J., 276–77
Butorphanol (Stadol), 126

caregiver's attitude (and child-birth
    experience), 269–84
  birth plan, 272–74
  caregiver's perspectives, 274–83
  caregiver's tips, 283–84
  changing attitude toward pain,
    270–71
  pain level rated accurately,
    271–72
Carroll, Ingrid, 278–79
Caton, Dr. Donald, 216, 228
cesarean delivery, 200–213
  complementary and alternative
    pain management, 213
  description of procedure, 200
  epidural and, 80, 92–94, 202
  general anesthesia and, 207–11
  pain relief and breast-feeding, 212
  pain relief used during procedure,
    201–11
  pain relief used during recovery,
    211–12
  reasons for, 201
  resources, 213
  partner's role, 205
  potential benefits, 205
  potential limitations, 206
  potential side effects, 206

potential side effects on new-born,
    207
  prescheduled (elective), 63–64,
    201
  spinal anesthesia (spinal block),
    202–7
Childbirth and Postpartum
    Professional Association, 23,
    185
childbirth fears, 52–71
  first-time moms, 54–58
  repeat moms, 59–64
  resources, 71
  stress factor, 64–71
Childbirth Without Fear (Dickead),
    226
Chritton, Laura, 111–12
clary sage, 187
codeine
  pain relief and breast-feeding after
    cesarean delivery, 212
combined spinal epidural (CSE),
    101–5
  conditions that may prevent use,
    104
  hospital, key questions to ask,
    109–10
  how it is done and feels, 101
  maternity unit size and, 6–7
  medications, 102
  partner and, 103
  potential benefits, 103–4
  potential limitations, 104
  potential side effects, 103
  reasons for choosing, 103
  sensation felt when CSE starts to
    work, 102
  what it is and does, 101
  when to use, 102
  See also epidural; patient-
    controlled epidural analgesia
complementary and alternative
    approaches (CAM), 137–99
  acupuncture, 140, 175–80
  aromatherapy, 140, 185–91
  birth ball, 141, 197–99
  Bradley Method, 140, 147–54

complementary and alternative
approaches (CAM) (*cont.*)
after cesarean delivery, 213
childbirth, how used during,
138–39
hypnotherapy, 140, 165–75
labor support, 140, 180–85
Lamaze, 140, 141–47
sterile water papules, 140,
191–94
transcutaneous electrical nerve
stimulation (TENS), 140,
194–96
water immersion, 140
Conception and Pregnancy (Goetzl),
274
Connor, Dr. Marsha, 179
Conrad, Laura, 149–50
Cron, Jennifer, 112–13

delivery nurse, 14–15
Dell, Dr. Diana, 58
Demerol (Meperidine), 125
desflurane, 209
Diazepam (Valium), 123
Dibal, Diedre A., 45–46
Dick-Read, Dr. Grantley, 225–26
domestic abuse as stress factor, 67
DONA International, 20–21, 22,
185
Donahue, Cheryl, 146–47
doula, 20–22
Downie, Jennifer, 152–53
Duramorph, 79, 205
dysmenorrhea (menstrual cramps),
39
dystocia, 38

Elizabeth (mother), 113–14
emotional abuse as stress factor, 67
environment, 3–23
anesthesiologist, 1517
birth center, 7–12
doula, 20–22
family physician, 20
hospitals, 4–7
labor and delivery nurse, 14–15
nurse-anesthetist, 17
nurse-midwife, 18–19
obstetrician, 13
professional midwife, 19
epi-doula, 22
epidural, 73, 74–100
breast-feeding success, 99–100
cesarean delivery and, 202
cesarean or instrumental delivery,
risk of, 80, 92–94, 97–98
conditions that may prevent use,
84
concerns and controversy,
92–100
headache, treating, 87
hospital, key questions to ask,
109–10
how it is done and feels, 75–79
labor, lengthening, 96
late in labor, 82–83
lower back pain, 95–96
maternity unit size and, 6–7
medications, physicians atempting
to dial down, 81–82
medications, potential side effects,
88–90
medications used, 79
newborn, potential side effects on,
90–92
oral intake and, 99
partner and, 85
patients on use of, 111–15
percent of women who use,
72
popularity of, 227
potential benefits, 86
potential limitations, 86–87
reasons for choosing, 83
sense of relief, 84–85
sensation felt when epidural kicks
in, 84
spiking a fever, 94–95
step by step, 77–78
what it is and does, 74–75
when to use, 80

See also combined spinal epidural;
patient-controlled epidural
analgesia
*Essential C-Section Guide: Pain
Control, Healing at Home, Getting
Your Body Back—and Everything
Else You Need to Know About a
Cesarean Birth, The* (Connolly/
Sullivan), 213
Essential Guide to Hysterectomy, The
(Streicher), 261

Fahnestock, Dr., 217
family physician, 20
Faris-Penn, Sheila, 172–73
Faye, Dr. Robyn, 243–45
fear. *See* childbirth fears
Fein, Biddy, 145
fentanyl, 126, 205, 209
fever spiking
epidural and, 94–95
Fisher, Shelly, 133–34
frankincense, 187

general anesthesia, 74
general anesthesia (cesarean delivery
and), 207–11
how it is done and feels, 208
how you may feel, 208–9
medications used, 209, 212
partner's role, 209
potential side effects (annoying
and unpleasant), 209
potential side effects (serious and
rare), 210
potential side effects on new-born,
211
what it is and does, 208
when used, 207
Goetzl, Dr. Laura, 274–75
Grubert, Dr., 216–17

Harmon, Linda, 141
Hartly, Tracy, 48

Harvard Medical School, 93
Hawkins, Dr. Joy, 48–49
high-risk pregnancy and bed rest,
66–67
hospitals, 4–7
epidural/spinal-epidural rates
according to maternity unit size,
6–7
pro and cons, 10–12
reasons to choose, 5
satisfaction rate, 7
Howe, Jennifer, 164
Husband-Coached Childbirth, 226
Hypnobabies Network, 175
hypnosis
Mesmeric pain relief, 216–17
hypnotherapy, 140, 165–75
caregiver's perspective, 170–71
concerns and controversy, 170
partner's role, 169
popularity of, 166
potential benefits, 169
potential limitations, 170
reasons for choosing, 169
research says, 189
resources, 175
what it is and does, 167–68
what women say, 171–75

ibuprofen
pain relief and breast-feeding after
cesarean delivery, 212
instrumental delivery
epidural and, 80, 97–98
isoflurane, 209

Joint Commission on Accreditation
of Healthcare Organizations
(JCAHO), 270

Keep, Nathan Cooley, 220
Kessler, Julia Lange, 46
Kosa, Jessica, 162–63
Kuppinger, Ellen, 150–51

labor nurse, 14–15
labor pain, 24–51
  back labor, 31
  books, 50–51
  cause of, 31–32
  common factors that impact,
    36–42
  description of, 29–30
  emotional response, 33–36
  intensity of, 25–27
  pain measurement scales, 32–33
  preparation, 42–50
  resources, 50
  stages of labor, 28–29
labor support, 140, 180–85
  caregiver's perspective, 184–85
  partner's role, 183
  potential benefits, 183
  potential limitations, 184
  research says, 184
  reasons for choosing, 182–83
  what it is and does, 180–81
Lacey, Theresa, 277–78
Lamaze, 140, 141–47
  caregiver's perspective, 145
  how it works and feels, 142–43
  partner's role, 144
  potential benefits, 144
  potential limitations, 144
  research says, 145
  resources, 147
  what women say, 145–47
  why women choose, 143–44
Lamaze, Dr. Fernand, 141, 227
Lamaze Organizations, 227
late-pregnancy loss as stress factor,
    65–66
lavender, 186
leeches (bloodletting)
  as pain relief, 217
Leopold, Prince, 219
Leupp, Constance, 222
Lidocane, 128
Listening to Mothers survey, 33–34
Lobel, Dr. Marci, 26
local anesthetic agents, 127–29
  commonly used, 128

potential benefits, 129
pudendal block, 128–29
potential side effects, 129
potential side effects on baby,
    129
what you may feel, 128–29
Longfellow, Fanny Appleton, 220
Lowe, Ananda, 275
Lowe, Dr. Nancy, 36
lower back pain
  cause of, 96
  epidural and, 95

Magner, Georgie Marks, 145–46
Maternity Center Association,
    33–34
Mather, Cotton, 216
McCubbin, Dr. James, 69
McGill Pain Questionnaire (MPQ),
    32–33
medications, 116–36
  analgesics, 124–27
  common types, 121
  local anesthetic agents, 127–29
  nitrous oxide, 129–33
  partner and, 119–20
  patients on use of, 133–36
  reasons to not choose, 118
  reasons to choose, 117
  sedatives, 121–23
menstrual cramps (dysmenorrhea),
    39
Meperidine (Demerol), 125
midazolam, 209
midwives
  nurse-midwife, 18–19
  professional midwife, 19
Midwives Alliance of North
    America, 19
Milo, Kimberley, 173–74
moms (and childbirth fears)
  first-time moms, 54–58
  repeat moms, 59–64
morphine, 125–26
moxibustion, 177
Muir, Holly, Dr., 110–11

Nalbuhine (Nubain), 126
narcotics, 125–26, 205
   pain relief and breast-feeding after
      cesarean delivery, 212
National Association of Child-
      bearing Centers, 7, 23
National Association of Holistic
      Therapy, 191
National Center for Complementary
      and Alternative Medicine, 180
National Commission for
      Certification of Acupuncture
      and Oriental Medicine, 179
National Organization for
      Competency Assurance
      (NOCA), 141
National Twilight Sleep Association,
   222–24
natural childbirth, 225–27
   Dr. Robert A. Bradley and,
      226–27
   Grantley Dick-Read and, 225–26
   Dr. Fernand Lamaze and, 227
neroli, 187
Nesacaine, 128
nitrous oxide, 129–33
   caregiver's perspective, 132–33
   how it is done and feels, 130
   potential benefits, 131
   potential limitation, 131
   potential side effects, 131
   potential side effects on baby, 131
   what it is and does, 130
   when to use, 130
Noll, Jill, 282
North American Registry of
      Midwives, 19
Nubain (Nalbuhine), 126
nurse-anesthetist, 17
nurse-midwife, 18–19
   percent of babies delivered by, 18

obstetrician, 13
Ogren, Carolyn, 280–82
Owen, Dr. Medge D., 264–68
Oxytocin (Pitocin), 39

pain measurement scales, 32–33
pain relief, 72–115
   combined spinal epidural (CSE),
      73–74, 101–5
   epidural, 6–7, 73, 74–100
   general anesthesia, 74
   patient-controlled epidural
      analgesia (PCEA), 105–10
pain relief (history of), 214–28
   ancient techniques, 216
   bloodletting (leeches), 217
   birthing stool, 217
   Dr. Donald Caton on, 216
   Mesmeric pain relief (hypnosis),
      216–17
   anesthesia, post, 219–28
   anesthesia, prior to, 215–19
   religious attitudes toward,
      217–19
Pan, Ho-Yu, 279–80
patient-controlled epidural analgesia
      (PCEA), 105–10
   caregiver's perspective, 110–11
   hospital, key questions to ask,
      109–10
   how it is done and feels, 106–7
   medications, 108
   partner and, 109
   potential benefits, 108
   potential limitations, 109
   potential side effects, 109
   sensation felt when PCEA is in
      place, 107–8
   what it is and does, 105–6
   when to use, 108
   See also epidural; combined spinal
      epidural
Patterson, Marcia, 44–45
Pearson, Kimberley, 174–75
peppermint, 187
Percocet
   pain relief and breast-feeding after
      cesarean delivery, 212
Perez, Paulina, 199
Pickens, Debbie, 43
Pitocin (Oxytocin), 39
Platt, Dr. Felicity, 132–33

pregnancy
  high-risk and bed rest, 66–67
previous miscarriage as stress factor,
  65–66
professional midwife, 19
propofol, 209

Ramus, Dr. Ronald, 49
Rehm, Dr. Ann, 233–35
Reiff, Jennie, 171–72
relaxation plan, 69–70
Riedmann, Gayle, 239–42
Roman chamomile, 187
rose oil, 187
Rosen, Dr. Mark, 132
Rush, Benjamin, 217

Schiavoni, Paula, 275–76
Secobarbital (Seconal), 123
Seconal (Secobarbital), 123
sedatives, 121–23
  potential benefits, 122
  potential side effects, 123
  potential side effects on baby,
    123
  Seconal (Secobarbital), 123
  Valium (Diazepam), 123
  what you may feel, 122
  when to use, 122
sevoflurane, 209
Shore, Donna, 135–36
Simkin, Penny, 21, 46–47
Simpson, James Young, 219, 220
Siverd, Amy, 114–15
Snow, John, 220
Society for Obstetric Anesthesia and
  Perinatology, 16–17
sodium pentothal, 209
Song, Marsha, 134–35
spinal anesthesia (cesarean delivery
  and), 202–7
  conditions that may prevent use,
    207
  how you may feel, 204–5
  medications used, 205

  reasons for, 205
  step by step, 203–4
  what it is and does, 202–4
spinal block. *See* spinal anesthesia
spinal epidural. *See* combined spinal
  epidural
Stadol (Butorphanol), 126
Stensland, Jude, 193–94
sterile water papules, 140, 191–94
  caregiver's perspective, 193–94
  how it is done and feels, 191–92
  partner's role, 192
  potential benefits, 193
  potential limitations, 193
  reasons for choosing, 192
  research says, 193
  resources, 194
  what they are and do, 191
  when to use, 192
Streicher, Dr. Lauren, 261–64
stress, 64–65
  abuse, domestic or emotional,
    67
  as health risk, 68
  high-risk pregnancy and bed rest,
    66–67
  managing, 68–70
  relaxation plan, 69–70
  previous miscarriage and late-
    pregnancy loss, 65–66

tokophobia, 58
Tracy, Marguerite, 222
transcutaneous electrical nerve
  stimulation (TENS), 140,
    194–96
  caregiver's perspective, 196
  how it is done and feels, 194–95
  partner's role, 195
  potential benefits, 195
  potential limitations, 195
  research says, 196
  resources, 196
  what it is and does, 194
  when to use, 195
Tuschhoff, Kerry, 170–71

Ulrich, Dr. Suzan, 255–58

Valium (Diazepam), 123, 209
Vaz, Heather, 153
Vicodin
    pain relief and breast-feeding after
        cesarean delivery, 212
Victoria, Queen, 221–22, 224

water immersion, 140, 154–65
    baby, risk to, 159–60
    birthing pools, 155
    caregiver's perspective, 162
    concerns and controversy, 159–62
    hospitals and, 154
    infection, risk of, 160
    pain relief, effectiveness of,
        161–62

partner's role, 157
potential benefits, 157
potential limitations, 157–59
research says, 160
resources, 165
what women say, 162–65
Walsh, Lisa, 43–44
What a Blessing She Had Chloroform:
    The Medical and Social Response
    to the Pain of Childbirth from
    1800 to the Present (Caton),
    228
Wiand, Nancy, 190
Wickersham, Rachel Dolan, 250–55
Wong, Dr. Cynthia A., 258–61
Woolfe, Virginia, 224

Zakowski, Dr. Mark, 230–32
Zuspan, Dr. Kathryn, 247–50

About the Authors

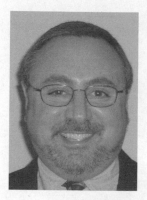

WILLIAM CAMANN, M.D., is the director of obstetric anesthesia at the Brigham and Women's Hospital in Boston, one of the most respected healthcare institutions in the world. Dr. Camann is also an associate professor of anesthesia at Harvard Medical School, and president of the Society for Obstetric Anesthesia and Perinatology. Dr. Camann is an internationally recognized authority on obstetric anesthesia and pain control during childbirth and has appeared on various local and national news programs including *The Today Show* with Katie Couric, *ABC World News Tonight,* and *Good Morning America.* He lives in Boston, Massachusetts.

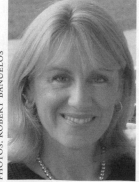

KATHRYN J. ALEXANDER, M.A., is a former child and family therapist and has worked in the healthcare field for over 15 years. Now a freelance writer, her work has appeared in many national parenting publications and on women's health websites. She is currently a contributing writer for *ePregnancy Magazine.* Ms. Alexander lives with her husband and two daughters in Charlotte, North Carolina.